NO EXCUSES

Building Better Bodies One Habit at a Time

Shaun Taylor Bevins PT, MPT

Transformation Press

I would like to dedicate this book to my children who continue to inspire me to live my best life. I would also like to thank my lifelong friend Heather Trout Osborne whose ongoing support in this venture has been invaluable and enduring. Finally, I would like to thank the entire No Excuses Facebook Community. The group, its members, and the entire experience have taught me so much about the challenges that people face when trying to take charge of their health. It has also been a source of ongoing inspiration and support for my own health and wellness journey.

Your body holds deep wisdom. Trust in it. Learn from it. Nourish it. Watch your life transform and be healthy.

BELLA BLEUE

CONTENTS

PREFACE

At the age of ten, I was thrilled to unwrap my first set of weights. At the age of thirteen, I joined my first gym. At eighteen, I started teaching group fitness. At twenty-two, I graduated with a Bachelor of Science in Nutritional Sciences, and at age twenty five, I followed up with a professional Master in Physical Therapy. Over the next two-and-a-half decades, I would continue my journey in health and fitness, both personally and professionally.

In January of 2020, a year many would later associate almost exclusively with COVID, I hosted an online fitness challenge. There were about fifty participants. The goal was to complete a 10-minute daily workout. Once the challenge ended, I decided to continue to support and promote the group with an intention of building a community that would foster healthy lifestyles via sustainable habits. At the time this book is being released, the No Excuses Facebook group has literally exploded to over 135,000 members worldwide, and it grows everyday.

The content of this book represents a lifetime of education, experience, and an ongoing passion for all that is healthy. In addition to my decades as a clinician, a fitness instructor, a wellness advocate, an educator, and even a writer, the information I share draws from over a hundred books on health and wellness, a number of which are referenced throughout the text.

What the book is not is a one-size-fits-all formula for success. Instead, I've attempted to share some of the wisdom and knowledge I've accumulated along the way with the hope that it will assist readers in finding their own path to success. It was a labor of love and one I embarked on with enthusiasm and determination. The book is only here because I showed up with a clear intention accompanied by action. Every. Single. Day. Week after week. Month after month. And even year after year.

Yet, for me, the real success of this project lies not in how well it is received or in its popularity among readers, but instead on its very existence. As a busy, full-time working mother of four, writing a book is not easy. Luckily, I applied the same principles and philosphy that I apply to my life and my wellness to this book. 80 percent of it was written in Google documents on my phone as I walked literally hundreds of miles over the course of two years. It is proof that process is everything, thinking outside the box is helpful, and consistency is key whether writing a book, achieving career success, or claiming the health and vitality we all long for.

Happy Reading and Best of Luck,
Coach Shaun

NO EXCUSES

Building Better Bodies One Habit at a Time

INTRODUCTION

"Why do you stay in the prison when the door is so wide open?"

RUMI

C elebrity icon Oprah Winfrey wowed her audience in the fall of 1988 when she strutted out onto the stage of The Oprah Winfrey Show, pulling a wagon of fat.

Sixty-seven pounds of fat to be exact—representing the weight she had recently shed on a liquid protein diet called Optifast. Before her reveal, Oprah had long struggled with her weight, tipping the scales in July of that same year at 212 pounds. So, it is no surprise that audiences were floored by the much slimmer and trimmer 145-pound version of the host, who looked exceptionally fit and fashionable in her stylish denim jeans and form-fitting black turtleneck.

If you happened to be around back then and watching like 18.4 percent of the households with televisions or 44 percent of the people tuned into their sets at the time the show aired, it was hard not to be impressed and a little envious.

Inspired by her success, over 200,000 viewers made a call to Optifast's manufactures (Sandoz Nutrition) after the show.

The fact that Oprah's triumph required twelve grueling weeks of a restrictive liquid protein diet (400 calories restrictive to be precise) did not deter viewers who were desperate to finally shed their own pesky pounds. Yet, just two weeks after the 26-week diet ended, sources reported Oprah had already gained back ten pounds.

I was a senior in high school at the time of Oprah's Optifast weight loss debut. I had yet to embark on my Bachelor of Science in Nutritional Sciences or my Professional Master in Physical Therapy. But I did understand the desire to be thin; to meet some arbitrary standard of beauty. And though only seventeen at the time, I had already been on my share of diets, desperate and willing to believe that the secret to the body of my dreams could be purchased for just $19.99.

Fast forward almost thirty-five years and not only is Oprah a little wiser, but so am I.

I wrote this book because I have spent the past three decades watching individuals not only struggling to take control of their weight and their health, like Oprah, but also failing to maintain that control long term.

Never have we had more trainers, health coaches, fitness influencers, paid and free YouTube workout channels, self-styled nutrition experts, weight-loss programs, fitness/food trackers, diet books, fitness challenges, supplements, pills, powders, lotions, and potions.

You name it, and we have packaged it, pedaled it, repackaged it, and re-pedaled it again under a different name.

So many "solutions" and yet many people are struggling to take control of their weight and their health. We are not only getting fatter, but we are also getting sicker. Lifestyle diseases like metabolic syndrome, type 2 diabetes, and heart disease —to name just a few—are not only on the rise but running rampant.

In 2019, approximately 1.4 million Americans died of the big three: heart disease, cancer, and diabetes.[1] And in 2017, a study commissioned by the American Diabetes Association and published in the March 2018 issue of *Diabetes Care* found that "for the cost categories analyzed, care for people with diagnosed diabetes accounts for 1 in 4 health care dollars in the U.S., and more than half of that expenditure [was] directly attributable to diabetes."[2]

Debilitating diseases like Alzheimer's and Parkinson's (both with links to lifestyle) are also increasing, while Covid outcomes are substantially worse in those who are obese.[3] And even for those vaccinated against the novel coronavirus, data has shown that comorbidities like heart disease and diabetes contribute to more serious illness if someone is infected.

Overweight and obesity and the behaviors contributing to overweight and obesity are a big part of the problem.[4]

Yet, even for those who shed some pounds, research suggests that, like Oprah, 95 percent of them will gain it back, the majority within two years, a chunk of them regaining *more* than what they lost.

Think about it. What other product with a 95 percent failure rate would you continue to buy?

Of course, this is exactly what people do: purchase a weight loss program, often repackaged or repurposed, but usually focused primarily on what people want: quick weight loss. And not merely quick. As of yesterday quick. And maybe they lose weight, or maybe they do not. But when all is said and done, the majority end up right back where they started, if they are fortunate enough to not regain more than they originally lost.

Only, they do not simply blame the trainer, the coach, or the pill, powder, or program. Despite their litany of excuses to suggest otherwise, they also blame themselves. And why not? They are the ones who fell off the wagon. They are the ones who stopped counting calories or macros. They are the ones who could not sustain getting up before dawn to squeeze in those grueling sweat fests. They are the ones who started making excuses.

It is not that their program was unsustainable; it is not because they neglected to learn and adopt effective long-term health strategies.

Many believe they are failures. And so, there stay stuck, until the next best-proven product or program comes along, and they convince themselves that this time will be different.

This time they are in it to win it. This time they have the right program. The right pill. The right powder. The right trainer. The right mindset. Or the right coach. This time they will not only succeed, but they will finally make that change they have always wanted. Once and for all.

So help them God.

Only we all know what happens. Of course, we do. It is why I wrote this book and why you are reading it.

Change is hard.

Real change takes time.

The only path to lasting change is through lasting change.

That is why I am not here to sell you the fitness fad of the hour or the current nutrition trend. You have tried those multiple times. Possibly with some success, but more likely than not failing long term.

This is because the problem does not necessarily lie with the diet, the trainer, the tracker, the coach, or the method. And it is not all your fault.

The real problem goes much deeper and encompasses so much more than any single weight loss modality on the market or personal shortcoming.

For most, it is a lack of consistency. One that is predictable but also inevitable. The weight loss industry has become masters at selling us exactly what we want: fast weight loss.

Yet, what they are not selling us—mainly because we are not buying—are long-term, sustainable strategies that, while effective, are just too damn slow for a world that expects instant everything.

This book is a compilation and fusion of what I have learned over the past thirty-plus years in the health and wellness industry, my clinical experience, and from my No Excuses Diet, Exercise, and Wellness Group on Facebook.

You will learn why consistency trumps intensity.

Why it is less about the nuances of the program and more about your ability to build lasting behaviors that support your goals, not just in the moment, but for the rest of your life.

In short, you will truly understand why slow and steady wins the race.

I cover the ins and the outs, the ups and the downs. The fads. The facts. The knowns and even the unknowns.

I hope that by sharing my accumulated knowledge and experience, you can make better-informed choices that are not simply focused on losing weight but on building a lean, strong, and healthy body over the long haul.

My reason—my why—for writing this book is to help others find long-term sustainable health and wellness strategies that not only work but that work long term. Instead, of before and after photos, I want you to have a forever photo, one that reflects the person you strive to be today and every day thereafter.

I am not dogmatic, and I have no vested interest in promoting any single wellness strategy. The truth is that while I can provide general guidelines and opinions based on my expertise and experience, only you can figure out what works for you at any given point. Like Keto? Okay. Intermittent fasting? If it works and works long term, then great. Need to count calories or macros? Knock yourself out.

There is no one-size-fits-all solution, but there are some basic and accepted universal ground rules that can get you started and keep you going.

When applicable, I provide the science because understanding why something works can increase compliance.

That said, you should not get bogged down in the details. There is no test at the end of this book. Instead, relax, read, learn, think, and enjoy with special emphasis on the enjoy part.

MINDSET MATTERS

"We cannot solve our problems with the same thinking we used when we created them."

ALBERT EINSTEIN

This Einstein quote hits the proverbial nail on its head. People do not necessarily fail at losing weight and getting fit because they are lazy, unwilling to work, or just do not want it enough. Lack of effort or commitment can certainly come into play. But a primary reason they fail is that they have flawed ideas about the problem and the solution.

They think the problem is their weight, their body fat, or another health metric gone wrong. And in one sense, they are right. Extra weight, too much fat relative to lean body mass, and poor health metrics can be a problem. But these things are not *the problem*. The root problem, or the first cause, is their lifestyle choices.

This distinction is important because you can lose weight, lean out, and get metrics within normal ranges in several ways, not all of them healthy and many of them unsustainable.

For example, let's pretend I have created a new weight loss program. Like Optifast's liquid diet, it is a little radical and very pricey, but ultra-effective and extremely quick. I lock you in a room (with your consent, of course) and carefully restrict your calories by intravenous feedings to a point that weight loss is inevitable (like a diet on steroids). I also have you perform a rigorous exercise program under the careful guidance and tutelage of our trainer to the stars, Fredrick, who pushes your body to lengths you thought unachievable. And eventually, much to your delight, you reach your goal.

So, I let you out, thank you for your time, and move on to my next customer while a much slimmer and even happier you return home to flaunt your new size *blank* (you-fill-in-the-blank) toned and beach-ready body.

But now what?

Initially, you manage. You attempt to eat your version of healthy as imperfect as it may be. You also do your best to mimic the grueling sweat sessions that are not the same without Fredrick standing over you. But as time passes, no longer strictly monitored, you fall back into old eating patterns. Without Fredrick there to push you, the frequency and intensity of your exercise sessions wane.

It does not happen overnight, but you gain weight back, pound by depressing pound. So, you restrict your calories and ramp up your sweat fests, hoping that is the answer. And, at first, it seems to work. Your weight gain slows. You might even drop a few of those regained pounds. Unfortunately, the weight returns even though you are eating less than ever.

While oversimplified, I hope you see where I am going with this. You had a problem: you were carrying some extra pounds. My groundbreaking program helped you solve that problem, albeit a little radically. And you left at your goal weight, a happy customer.

Problem solved, right?

Wrong!

The strategy you employed to lose the weight was not sustainable or practical over the long term. And while my program delivered on its promise to get you the body of your dreams at record speed, it ultimately failed because you gained the weight back.

What you did not realize or neglected to acknowledge is that to solve the problem, you needed to change the forces that created the problem in the first place and not just for a few weeks or a few months.

Unfortunately, the assumption that a calorie surplus is the sole cause of weight gain is not only naïve, but it is also wrong. This does not mean that calories do not matter—they do—but instead that many other things matter as much as or even more.

The problem was never your weight. It was your behavior. And while my calorie deficit solution (decreased calorie consumption, increased calorie expenditure) resulted in weight loss, it did nothing to address why were you eating so many calories in the first place. Remember, the body is designed to thrive and sustain the status quo. There are a multitude of feedback loops in place to keep the machine healthy and working well.

What went wrong?

The answer to this question is more complicated than the calories in versus calories out equation suggests.

For example, thanks to studies conducted by Dr. Satchin Panda, who summarized his findings in *The Circadian Code*, we have evidence that when we eat may be as important as both how much we eat and what.

We also have research suggesting the quality of calories and the way they affect insulin can influence both weight and weight gain.

Increases in ghrelin, a make-you-hungry hormone secreted by the gut in response to an empty stomach or a calorie deficit, may also be important as it stays elevated long after we stop restricting calories. This increase in ghrelin leads to an increase in hunger that persists long after the diet ends.

Resistance to leptin, ghrelin's counterpart and a satiety hormone that tells us when to stop eating, is another possible contributing factor. Produced by adipose tissue, leptin tells our brain that we have eaten enough. However, those with large deposits of fat (which is not simply inert tissue but an endocrine organ) may produce too much leptin. Over time, this can lead to leptin resistance. No longer sensitive to the leptin circulating in the bloodstream, we continue to eat although we have had more than enough.

There are other factors we will touch on throughout this book, but rather than overwhelm you now, I want to draw attention to the simple fact that it is never as simple as we think. Sometimes the obvious solution is not the right one.

Just because something works short term does not mean it will work long term. What we think works and what works may be at odds.

Even the way we frame the solution matters and may require us to rethink the process. For example, as illustrated in the chart below, there can be a huge difference between simply losing weight and building a lean, strong, and healthy body. One is simply focused on the scale at all costs while the other is focused on promoting health. The latter is clearly more important as it supports the former.

Losing Weight	Building a Lean, Strong, Healthy Body
Defines success using a negative term that implies loss	Defines success by using a positive term that implies creating something of value
Ties success to weight as opposed to body composition	Implies building muscle and/or losing fat
Does not necessarily require long-term behavior change	Requires long-term behavior change
Tends to be more outcome	Tends to be more process

oriented	oriented
Does not necessarily connect the outcome to health and behaviors that support health	Connects outcome to health
A maintenance phase is implied but because core issues are not necessarily addressed, many people struggle after the weight is lost	There is no difference between the active phase and the maintenance phase. The maintenance phase is an extension of the active loss phase.
Often results in a cycle of yo-yo dieting	Builds sustainable habits that support leanness
Focus is on thinness but not necessarily fitness	Both leanness and fitness are emphasized

Summary

Solving a problem often requires a shift in our thinking about both the problem and the solution. When it comes to getting leaner (losing fat and/or gaining muscle as opposed to just losing weight), it is important to understand that weight is not the problem. Poor lifestyle choices and habits that do not support our desired level of leanness and health are. Therefore, if we want to get leaner, we need to shift the focus from weight loss achieved primarily through an obsession with temporary calorie deficits (yes, calories matter but not nearly as much as or in the way we think) to a focus on mastering long-term behaviors that support health and leanness over the long haul. We need to become experts at eating a healthy, sustainable, and inclusive diet, moving regularly in ways that feel good and support our body, getting adequate sleep, and managing stress.

Take Home Point:

Building a lean, strong, and healthy body often requires that we re-evaluate and rethink our attitudes about health, weight, and weight loss.

"Instant gratification is not soon enough."

MERYL STREEP

Whoever said good things come to those that wait lacked Jeff Bezos' vision or could not comprehend the pure joy of eating a stress-free, mess-free take-out meal from your favorite restaurant.

Let's face it. Not all good things require waiting. Likewise, *quick and fast* does not always imply poor quality, either. Yet, while Amazon has done its part to prove otherwise, there are still some things that cannot be same-day delivered or shipped overnight.

Some good things really do take time. And not only do they take time, but they also rarely provide an immediate return on investment. And that has always been tough, but especially today when instant gratification has become the expected norm.

Losing weight or getting fit is one of those things that cannot be purchased hassle-free or delivered via *Prime*. And this is a problem because not only do we want to see results as of yesterday, but we also want to see results every day, and we want our package—the body of our dreams—to appear much like our Amazon orders.

And therein lies one of the biggest challenges we face. Our need to see immediate and regular, if not daily, progress toward our goal (usually defined by three arbitrary numbers on the scale) is sometimes the very thing that keeps us from seeing the results we crave.

Many of us intuitively know. Most of us have been warned. The scale lies. Memes about the scale's shortcomings are not only common and funny, but they are also true. Weight can fluctuate throughout the month, the week, the day, and even the hour. And this is because so many things can affect our gravitational pull. Monthly cycles, water retention, an undigested meal, bloating, and dehydration to name just a few.

But it goes deeper than that. Most scales do not tell us anything about body composition, and the scales that claim to (the ones that tell us body fat) are known for huge margins of error. Readings cannot only be inaccurate, but they can also vary from day to day.

And yet, too many of us put way too much emphasis on what that scale says.

I often joke with friends, patients, and clients that were I to sneak into their bathroom and rig their scale to read ten pounds lighter, not only would the person they see in the mirror look thinner, but their pants would also fit looser, their mood would be better, and they might even walk straighter and with more confidence throughout the day.

But this brief experiment would also work in the opposite direction. If I instead rigged their scale to read ten pounds heavier, their reflection would look heavier, their pants might fit tighter, their mood might be lower, and they might walk through their day feeling defeated and like a failure.

Such is the power of our thoughts.

It is also why tying our success to those three arbitrary numbers and expecting immediate, daily results can set us up for disappointment and failure, not necessarily physically, since we know the scale lies, but mentally because even though we know the scale lies, we still crave reinforcement that we are making progress. That all our sweat fests and salads, all our food prep and Fitbit steps have not been in vain.

Yet, this is a flawed strategy that may or may not serve us at any moment. Some days, the scale may reward us, and others not so much. And we could view it as a wash if perceived failure were not more heavily weighted than a comparable perceived success. Thanks to our risk-averse brains—which evolved to avoid danger—we fear failure more than we enjoy success. If life were a video game, perceived failures would penalize us ten points while perceived successes would earn us a measly plus one.

Failure not only hurts, but it really hurts. And while success can feel good, it rarely feels as good as failure feels bad.

While it is tempting to preach the merits of patience, the desire to see progress is understandable. To seek validation for our efforts is the most natural thing in the world. Unfortunately, the scale is a poor, inconsistent form of validation that has the potential to do more harm than good. This does not mean we should not ever weigh ourselves, but that we should read the display with a grain of salt, aware that what we see is not necessarily a reflection of our true progress.

Our measurements, the way our clothes fit, and even blood tests provide more objective and meaningful feedback, however, even these measurements have limitations. And this is because the actual goal should not be a certain weight, a certain size, or a certain lab marker but a mastering of the behaviors that support that weight, that size, and that lab marker long term.

Any measurement, no matter how objective, ties to one moment in time. And just as failure is not fatal, success is not final. Things like weight, body fat, blood pressure, and fasting blood sugar are all temporary and will change to reflect our behaviors in the present.

Input equals output. Change input temporarily and output changes temporarily. But to change output permanently, you must change input permanently.

For this reason, success should not be tied to something as transient and arbitrary as three numbers on a scale or even some of these other metrics, but instead to our ability to master and adopt the behaviors that support our long-term health and wellness goals.

Success is not weighing xxx on the scale. It is consuming more fruits and veggies. Prioritizing sleep. Eating more whole food and less processed food, especially added sugar. Moving daily in ways that feel good but that challenge the body a little and that also help maintain the entire machine. Fasting at least twelve hours to support gut health, etcetera. In a nutshell, success is not in achieving the grand outcome, but in mastering the tiny details that support that outcome.

That kind of change takes time. Real time.

Summary

In a world of instant gratification, it is understandable that we crave instant results. It is also natural to seek validation to know that all our hard work is paying off. Unfortunately, using progress toward our goal as determined by the scale or even some other more objective measurement misses the mark. The outcome is transient. It is the process—those set of behaviors that support the desired outcome—that needs to be mastered. Therefore, our success/progress should relate to our ability to follow through and adopt those behaviors.

Take Home Point:

To build a lean, strong, and healthy body, we should tie success to mastering sustainable behaviors that support a lean, strong, and healthy body over the lifespan. Period. End of story.

"The secret to getting ahead is getting started."

MARK TWAIN

Start where you are, use what you have, and do what you can. Always.

But get started. And then keep going by building skills that support your desired outcome through daily practice.

Note, I did not say strict adherence or perfection, an expectation that often leads to failure. I said practice.

Ironically, getting fit and losing weight and/or getting healthy is one of the few skills we expect to master immediately. We accept that once we have decided to lose weight or improve our health, all that we need is motivation and determination. And while motivation and determination are assets, what most of us need is practice—daily consistent practice at making choices that support our long-term goals.

You become a better soccer player by practicing those skills that make you a better soccer player. You advance in your job by mastering those skills that make you good at your job. You become better at any skill through repeated and regular practice.

And if you want to master behaviors that support a lean, strong, and healthy body, then you must practice those behaviors.

Practice assumes that you have not already mastered a skill, or if you have, you are fine-tuning it or training to sustain it.

The same applies to a particular lifestyle choice and life in general. And while practice does not always make perfect, it usually leads to progress.

A major component of building a lean, strong, and healthy body is practice. The majority of us have not mastered those behaviors that support the desired outcome. Practice not only improves the skills needed to reach and sustain our health and wellness goals, but eventually those skills become second nature and automatic. They become a habit.

But that takes time. So, too often, we exchange an illusion of progress (quick weight loss fixes) for actual progress (mastering those behaviors that support long-term change).

Want to eat better? Practice eating better. Plan meals. Work on incorporating more fruits and veggies into your diet. Start looking at food labels and ingredients and then choosing those foods that are healthiest (least processed) the majority of the time. Experiment with increasing the overnight fast to improve gut health.

Want to exercise more and improve your fitness? Start practicing regular daily movement with a respect for where your body is in the moment. That means choosing movements that support health and fitness and do not lead to injury because you pushed too hard or too soon.

Most importantly, practice patience. Building a lean, strong, and healthy body takes time. And you might not always see the desired progress, which is slow, but more sustainable and long-lasting.

Again, real and lasting change requires real and lasting change. This not only takes time and practice, but it also takes being honest with yourself about what you will do and do long term to support your goals. You must understand that all levels of fitness and leanness require a level of commitment to a set of behaviors that support that fitness and leanness.

The time investment and level of commitment to nutrition and exercise needed to sustain 18 percent body fat differ from what is required to support 25 percent body fat.

Likewise, if your motivation is simply to get healthier, your forever program may look quite different from someone who has specific fitness or performance goals.

Input equals output. Your desired output—or goal—determines the input needed to reach and sustain that goal.

Unfortunately, the fitness industry often treats everyone as if they are at the same starting point with the same resources and also as if they share a common destination. Yet this is a huge and potentially dangerous assumption. I cannot tell you how often someone has ended up on my treatment table because they started a new one-size-fits-all program that was not even in alignment with their goals.

That said, regardless of your desired output, being consistent with the required input takes practice. Even when mastered, these skills, though they may become second nature, still require reinforcement through ongoing practice or regular participation.

We are what we repeatedly do. Amen!

Summary

Starting is hard. But starting is only the first challenge we face. Continuing to go is just as hard, if not harder. Quick fixes often promote quick weight loss by promoting strategies that are impractical and unsustainable long term. The actual key is to master and reinforce behaviors that support our goals both in the short and the long term. And this always requires practice, a considerable time investment, and even failure. Unfortunately, there is no way around addressing those long-term behaviors.

Take Home Point:

To build a lean, strong, and healthy body you must practice those behaviors that support your desired outcome, understanding that perfection is often unrealistic but that over time you will get better, things will get easier, and the slow progress you see will build on itself. Little gains eventually become big gains.

"Success is the product of daily habits, not once-in-a-lifetime transformations."

JAMES CLEAR, ATOMIC HABITS

The above quote is just one of many gems on the power of habit that James Clear includes in his book *Atomic Habits*, which I highly recommend.

It is easy to be wowed by the transformation stories of others. It is why *before and after* photos have become a staple in the marketing campaigns of so many fitness programs and products alike. And with good reason. What could be a better advertisement for whatever it is you are selling than a real-life success story? And thanks to social media, they are everywhere, tempting us with promises of success that say if this average person can do it, so can you.

The problem is that they never show us the after-after photo. After the program is over, after the diet is done, after the weight is lost. They do not show us where this person is in a year or two when, unable to sustain the calorie deficits, dietary restrictions, and grueling workout regimens, they have regained most if not all the weight.

Not that everyone who loses weight will regain it. But unfortunately, many will. And this is not because the program does not promote weight loss. Clearly, the program worked as advertised. The problem is many programs are unsustainable, and they are unsustainable because, by design, they produce weight loss and usually quick weight loss. What they fail to do is maximize long-term compliance.

In the fitness industry's defense, they are giving us—the consumer—exactly what we want even if they know it is not what we need. And trust me, when a fitness guru tries to give consumers what they need, they rarely sell many programs.

Gradual weight loss that will take time and consistency and a lifelong commitment just cannot compete with *transform your body in twelve weeks or less, meal plans and workouts included, $69.99 with a money-back guarantee.*

Ironically, most people know they need to make a lifestyle change, only they fail to embrace exactly what that means.

Let me make it simple. It means forever!

A lifestyle change requires permanently replacing old habits that do not support our goals with new ones that do. And that takes time and effort. It also involves a healthy dose of failure and a return on investment that makes the tortoise in the famous Aesop's fable look like a cheetah in comparison. Slow is often an understatement, especially by today's standards. And we do not like slow. We do not like to wait. And with weight loss, we are even less willing to wait.

We also overestimate our ability to stay compliant. We forget that real life is a series of trials and tribulations, and that fickle thing we call motivation will wane or lose out to other competing motivations. Thus, we not only need a solid long-term strategy, but also one that is flexible.

Another common mistake is underestimating the time necessary to establish new habits, as well as forgetting that old habits are like clingy ex-lovers who, wanting us back, are waiting patiently in the wings with open arms to console us when things get a little rocky in our new relationship.

Now, I am not trying to scare you. Though forming new habits can be tough, it can and is done all the time. Still, the inability to adopt habits that support our long-term goals is one of the biggest reasons we struggle to lose weight or lose it but then gain it back.

Of course, there are other factors at play. For example, prolonged periods of strict calorie restriction with the end goal of creating calorie deficits can cause our metabolism to slow down via a whole slew of biological feedback loops that once kept us from starving to death in a world where food was not available on every street corner 24/7. So, even if we can stick to the diet long term, we may find that we need to eat less and less to maintain thanks to our body's willingness and ability to adapt.

And there are other potential factors such as injuries that result from fitness programs not well suited to the individual, as well as major life events that not only throw us a curveball but the whole damn ballpark.

Yet, most times it comes down to a focus on the transformation, which is temporary, instead of the vehicle for true and lasting transformation, which are the habits that support that transformation long term.

Complete books, like the one referenced at the beginning of this chapter, explore habit, and I cannot do the topic justice in this book. That said, habit, aka our daily behaviors, is a big part of building and maintaining a lean, strong, and healthy body.

Summary

While it is easy to be seduced by the idea of transformation, it is important to remember that transformation is nothing more than the product of our daily habits. Every man and woman who succeeds may not have a supportive spouse or family member behind them, but they all have supportive habits working for them. So, think big, but act small. First, ask yourself *what daily behaviors will support my goals and my transformation?* Are they sustainable not just for a few weeks or months but for forever and ever, amen? If so, get busy and start practicing. The more you practice said behaviors, the more likely they are to become habitual, meaning they require little thought and/or motivation. For lack of a better word, they move on autopilot. And what a beautiful thing it is when our habits support our goals because that is where real transformation lives.

Take Home Point:

Building a lean, strong, and healthy body requires that

we practice behaviors that support our goals. With enough practice and repetition and even a little luck, those behaviors become habits. Establishing good habits is the key to a successful and lasting transformation.

"Motivation is what gets you started. Habit is what keeps you going."

JIM ROHN

In my No Excuses Facebook group, people often ask about motivation: how to find it, how to keep it, and/or how to overcome a lack of it. What they do not always realize is that we are always motivated. It is just sometimes our motivation to do something that feels good in the moment but that does not support our long-term goals trumps our motivation to do something that supports our long-term goals but that does not feel so good in the moment.

And so, it is not a lack of motivation that keeps us from following through. Instead, it is a powerful motivation to do what feels good at a specific time that wins out over our more general but weaker motivation to make lasting change.

And this is true of any goal we set, lifestyle or otherwise.

This is another reason developing good habits is so important. Habits are not at the mercy of motivation. By definition, habits are those behaviors that require little effort or motivation. As stated previously, they are our autopilot setting. That is what makes them so powerful.

Unfortunately, what motivates us to act at any given point is hard to predict, let alone control, and why motivation seems like such a fickle thing.

Think about it. The motivation to sleep in promises your body an immediate reward, whereas getting up to exercise may not only feel like a punishment but the reward is often delayed. It is a no-brainer. Sure, sheer determination and willpower may win a few battles, at least initially, but these attributes are finite resources in limited supply.

The reality is you do not need more motivation. You need to

minimize the need for motivation.

For example, think about your current habits and just how hard they are to break. And that is a good thing if those habits also support your goals.

It is also why building better habits through practice is the ticket to realizing your desires. The road to hell may be paved with good intentions and reliance on motivation in the moment, but the road to success is paved with good habits.

Repeat after me. *We are what we repeatedly do.*

We are not what we want to do. We are not what we think we should do. We are not even what we occasionally do when divine inspiration strikes. Yet, we are the sum of our daily actions, most of them habitual.

So, if you think you lack motivation, think again. You have plenty of motivation. What you need are better habits.

Summary

That we lack motivation is a fallacy. The inability to follow through with certain behaviors has nothing to do with a lack of motivation. It is the exact opposite. We always have motivation, only sometimes it is motivation to do what feels good in the moment as opposed to what serves us long term. The problem with depending on motivation is that what motivates us at any point in time, like sleeping in or indulging in a delicious piece of cake, may be stronger than our watered-down motivation to lose weight, exercise, or make better food choices. That is why developing better habits is so crucial to long-term success.

Take Home Point:

If you want to build a lean, strong, and healthy body, you need better habits and not necessarily more motivation.

"Success is neither magical nor mysterious. Success is the natural consequence of consistently applying the fundamentals."

JIM ROHN

Up to this point, I have covered the most common mindset mistakes I see people make when it comes to expectations. And I have done so because in thirty-plus years of doing this, I have learned that our attitudes and beliefs about the process are crucial to our success. Unfortunately, we often expect too much too soon, being unrealistic about not only what it takes but how long it takes. We get seduced by the quick fix, even though deep down we know quick fixes do not work long term.

We want to believe that if we can simply stay motivated, we can accomplish anything, only motivation is not reliable.

We also tie success to the scale rather than those long-term behaviors that support our health and wellness goals, not just in the moment, but over the long haul. And we forget that mastering those behaviors requires practice and repetition.

So, in case you missed them, let me summarize some key points before moving on:

- Lasting change requires making lasting change
- Real and lasting change takes time
- Most weight loss strategies/programs were designed to produce fast weight loss, not to build and sustain lean, strong, and healthy bodies
- Studies have shown that 95 percent of people who lose weight will gain it back within a few years
- Consistency will always trump intensity
- Weight is never the problem but a symptom of another problem

- We should link success to building long-term and sustainable behaviors that support a lean, strong, and healthy body, not an arbitrary and temporary metric like weight, body fat, or some other physiologic assay
- Input equals output—change input temporarily and you change output temporarily, but change input permanently and you change output permanently
- Changing input takes practice
- Practice builds habit
- Habit keeps us going when motivation cannot

So, with that out of the way, we can shift our focus to the fundamentals, a set of behaviors that support a lean, strong, and healthy body. This is where my book may diverge from someone else's book, as I am going to share my formula for success.

While there are no one-size-fits-all approaches to building lean, strong, and healthy bodies, there are proven strategies that not only support leanness but that also support health. When implemented consistently, these behaviors not only get you started, but they keep you moving—and moving continuously—in the right direction.

The strategies I recommend not only have a basis in science but also draw from my three decades of experience.

They are not new. They are not radical or revolutionary. They are not restrictive. And they are certainly no secret. You have probably already heard about them before.

They are often common sense. Always practical. Most importantly, they are sustainable and effective.

Of course, they do not represent the only path to success. But if you are completely at a loss for where to begin, they can provide a sound foundation from which to build your dream body.

So, let's get started.

EAT BETTER, WORKOUT SMARTER

E xactly how does one eater better, not less and workout smarter, not harder? Well, the answer depends on whom you ask. My answer (not calorie restriction) is based on my education, my personal and professional experience, my continuing studies, and to some extent, even my beliefs. It is informed by science but also reflects my interpretation of that science as applied to real-life scenarios as I have experienced them.

For practical purposes, I try to keep it simple.

1. Eat 7-8 servings of fruits and veggies every day
2. Try to limit added sugars to under 35 grams a day
3. Increase the overnight fast to a minimum of 12 hours
4. Eat whole healthy foods at least 80 percent of the time
5. Learn how to indulge responsibly and guilt-free
6. Move on most days in ways that feel good and challenge your body a little in some way
7. Implement a comprehensive fitness program that addresses all areas of fitness, including cardiovascular fitness, muscular fitness (strength and endurance), mobility and flexibility, as well as balance and coordination
8. Get 7-8 hours of quality sleep on most nights

Simple? Yes.

Easy? Not always.

Sustainable? If you build good habits.

Ironically, when you do these things, calories, macros, fiber, protein, probiotics, vitamins, minerals, and phytonutrients—all those things the pseudo-experts tell us to worry about and count—often take care of themselves.

"The bottom line is that the human body is complex and subtle, and oversimplifying-as common sense sometimes impels us to do-can be hazardous to your health."

ANDREW WEIL

We have most certainly made living a healthy lifestyle harder than it needs to be.

But simplifying a process for practical purposes differs from oversimplifying the underlying mechanisms that are at work.

For example, I can teach a child how to throw a baseball and throw it effectively without undermining, diminishing, or invoking the physics behind it. Interestingly, while the physics involved in throwing a baseball has not changed, our understanding of it has, just as our understanding of weight and weight gain has changed and evolved.

There are many theories about our weight. The most basic and most ingrained is the calories in versus calories out model of weight gain and weight loss. Eat more than you burn, and you gain weight. Eat less than you burn, and you lose. Get it just right and you stay the same.

Pretty simple, right?

Wrong!

Like most oversimplifications, this theory ignores other contributing and confounding factors.

While too many calories contribute to weight gain and though calorie deficits do lead to weight loss, it turns out it is a lot more nuanced than that.

Unless you have access to sophisticated equipment and track, log, and measure all movement and food, the calories in and calories out are just an estimation based on an estimation, often based on an estimation. And that is an awful lot of estimating.

The calories in versus calories out model also assumes the body is a closed system. But we know this is not true.

For example, the timing of your meal and the quality of the calories can affect the insulin response, which can influence calorie absorption and storage.

Calorie deficits can also lead to increases in the hunger hormone ghrelin, which persists even after the restriction is over. This means you continue to feel hungry even though you are no longer cutting back, and hunger plays a significant role in overeating.

Stress, lack of sleep, and hormonal fluctuations can also affect hunger and satiety while influencing energy storage and mobilization.

Calories eaten too close to bedtime move through the gut sluggishly, which can affect the rate and number of calories absorbed.

The gut microbiome—the tiny little bugs that live in our gastrointestinal tract—may also play a factor in how our body processes calories.

Weight, body composition, age, sex, hormonal health, and level of fitness can all impact the number of calories burned both at rest and during exercise and non-exercise movement.

The body can also make up for an increase in calories burned during exercise by causing a spontaneous though observed decrease in non-exercise/movement calories burned, which differs from and may be in addition to a reduction in BMR (basal metabolic rate or calories burned at rest).

Weight loss, which sometimes includes muscle, not only affects metabolism, but it lowers your energy needs during waking hours because you are carrying less weight around.

And while calorie deficits often lead to weight loss in the short term, for whatever reason, they do not seem to work long term. Even if you do not accept the statistic that 95 percent of people who lose weight gain it back, and even if scientists do not understand exactly why, I would bet most of you know firsthand the shortcomings of the diet culture built around the calories in versus calories out model, or you would not be reading this book.

And YES, in theory, calories DO matter, and calorie deficits can assist with weight loss. But from a practical standpoint, the calorie deficit approach to getting leaner does not provide a clear and effective plan of attack that works in both the short and long term. It also results in physiological and psychological changes that favor weight regain as beautifully described in a science brief written by Traci Mann, professor of psychology and author of *Secrets from the Eating Lab: The Science of Weight Loss, the Myth of Willpower and Why You should Never Diet Again.* The brief is published on the American Psychological Association site.[5] (I've read the book, too, and it is worth a read.)

In theory, the goal would be to eat as much as you can and move as little as possible and still reach and maintain your ideal weight. Basically, eat better, not less and workout smarter, not harder. That is the strategy for which I advocate and serves as a premise for the specific behaviors I recommend.

For more reading on the shortcomings of the calories in versus calories out model I recommend *The Circadian Code* by Satchin Panda, *The Obesity Code* and *The Diabesity Code* by Dr. Jason Fung, *The Calorie Myth* by Jason Bailor, *How Not to Diet* by Michael Greger, *The Belly Fat Effect* by Mike Mutzel, *Why You Eat What You Eat* by Rachel Herz, *Real Food, What to Eat and Why* by Nina Planck, *Always Hungry* by David Ludwig, and *The Hungry Brain* by Stephan Guyenet.

"We should all be eating fruits and vegetables like our lives depended on it, because they do."

DR. MICHAEL GREGER

Multiple decades doing this and the best piece of advice I can give when asked about ways to improve a diet is to eat more fruits and veggies. And once you do, eat even more.

Loaded with vitamins and minerals essential to normal growth and development, fruits and veggies really are gifts from the gods They contain powerful phytochemicals like polyphenols, flavonoids, and carotenoids that not only prevent disease but have a role in curing it. They provide an important source of fiber that not only promotes our health but that also feeds the important microbes that live in our gut and that are major players in both health and disease.

The scientific literature contains a tremendous amount of research supporting their benefits, and yet my experience has been that most people are not getting enough. In fact, according to the CDC, only 1 in 10 adults consumes the minimal 1.5-2 cups of fruits and 2-3 cups of veggies per day recommended by federal guidelines.[6]

If there is something that continually surprises me, it is how little produce most people eat.

Besides their multitude of health benefits, fruits and veggies are nutrient-dense and low in calories, which means not only are they filling but you get a boatload of nutrition at a very low-calorie cost. They are about as close to the perfect food as we can get.

For this reason, I recommend eating at least 7-8 combined servings of fruits and veggies a day and, whenever possible, eating the rainbow. This will enhance the overall diversity of nutrients in your diet.

Though serving sizes vary, a serving of vegetables is roughly one cup of raw or cooked veggies or two cups of leafy greens, and a serving of fruit is one cup of raw or cooked fruit.

Aren't fruits bad because they contain sugar?

Unfortunately, this myth has gained way too much traction thanks to pseudo-experts in the fitness industry that do not understand the chemistry of food. Though fruit does contain fructose naturally, it is an unconcentrated source, unlike the fructose-containing added sweeteners such as high fructose corn syrup, which have been intentionally concentrated.

And while fruits have a high glycemic index (which measures how quickly blood sugar rises after consumption), they have much lower glycemic loads (a more accurate reflection of the true rise in blood sugar because it addresses typical serving size).

Of course, if you have type 2 diabetes, meaning you are metabolically sick and your body no longer recognizes insulin, you might want to focus more on vegetables, stick to wild berries, and other fruits with lower glycemic indexes, or pair fruit with other foods that contain fat, protein, and complex carbohydrates to slow down digestion. We will talk more about type 2 diabetes later, but for now, I will just point out that according to the **American Diabetic Association**, a healthy diabetic diet can and should include fruits and veggies.

What about juicing and/or blending in smoothies?

Unlike blending fruits and veggies in smoothies where you will still consume the entire product, juicing strips away important nutrients like fiber. That said, given that most people are drinking other nutrient-void and sometimes sugar-laden beverages, juicing is a healthier option. Just be sure that if you are juicing, you are still eating intact fruits and veggies at other times during the day.

What about organic?

The answer to this question will depend on whom you ask. While locally and organically grown food is a slightly superior product regarding nutrition and taste and arguably more environmentally friendly, many experts believe that eating more fruits and veggies, organic or not, is worthwhile.

If, however, you are worried about exposure to pesticides, there are basic steps you can take to minimize your exposure and expense.

To begin with, according to the Environmental Working Group, a nonprofit dedicated to clean living, a significant percentage of the pesticides used are applied to a small percentage of crops. Every year they release two lists: *The Dirty Dozen* and *The Clean Fifteen*. Foods on the dirty list are the most likely to contain pesticide residue, while foods on the clean list are the least likely.[7]

Another strategy is to eat a diversity of fruits and veggies to limit exposure to any one pesticide.

Fresh versus frozen versus canned?

While fresh is certainly the most popular, frozen can be a great alternative, particularly if used in smoothies. Most frozen produce is harvested at peak ripeness and flash frozen, making it nutritionally sound. Canned foods may or may not be as healthy since many are packed in syrup with added sugars to enhance flavor or with sodium to prevent bacterial growth. Exposure to BPA from cans may also be a concern.

I am not sure I can eat that many servings. What should I do?

First, start where you are. If you are currently eating 1-2 servings a day, increasing it to 7-8 is unrealistic and even intimidating. Instead, shoot for 2-3 and work from there.

Tips for Eating More Fruits and Veggies

1. Add fruits and veggies to your current staples whenever possible, and it is always possible. A slice of avocado to a sandwich, sautéed mushroom, onions, and fresh spinach to a burger, and a can of pumpkin to your tomato sauce.
2. Build your meal around a fruit and/or veggie base. So, rather than eating veggies as a side with your chicken and rice, eat chicken and rice as a side with your veggies.
3. Keep a bowl of fruit on your counter where it is easily accessible.
4. Have cut and ready-to-go veggies in the fridge where they are easy to see and reach.
5. Commit to eating at least two servings of fruits and/or veggies with every meal.
6. Read about the various health benefits of fruits and veggies to get you excited about eating them.

"Everybody's got their poison, and mine is sugar."

DERRICK ROSE

It seems unfair that something that tastes so good to us should be so bad for us. Yet, the evidence is mounting. Added sugars are not simply benign empty calories. Too much added sugar is detrimental to our health.

Added sugars lead to chronic systemic inflammation, a common contributing factor to lifestyle diseases like heart disease, high blood pressure, Alzheimer's, and cancer.

Added sugar can also accelerate aging thanks to AGEs (advanced glycation end products) which are harmful free radicals that form when sugar in your bloodstream attaches to proteins. And because most added sugars are a concentrated source of fructose, a monosaccharide that the liver must metabolize, it contributes to non-alcoholic fatty liver disease.

Insulin, a catabolic hormone that promotes fat storage, can spike in response to the ingestion of simple added sugars. If substantial and frequent, these insulin spikes contribute to insulin resistance, which can cause diabetes, metabolic syndrome, and weight gain. In *Nature Wants Us to Be Fat,* Dr. Richard Johnson suggests that eating the large quantities of fructose found in added sugars can increase the risk of metabolic diseases like type 2 diabetes and metabolic syndrome even in the absence of excessive weight gain.

Though some added sugar in the diet is benign, too much and too often may literally kill us. The revised 2020-2025 US Dietary Guidelines recommends that adults and children over the age of two limit added sugars to less than 10 percent of their calorie intake. For an adult who eats 2000 calories, this would equate to only 200 calories from added sugar or fifty grams.[8] The AHA (American Heart Association) goes even further. They encourage women to limit added sugars to under 100 calories or twenty-five grams/day and men to under 150 calories or thirty-five grams/day.[9]

While fifty grams of added sugar sounds significant, it is the proverbial drop in the bucket when you consider a can of cola sold in the US has about forty grams.

The data is clear. Too much added sugar is bad for us, and we are eating way too much.

On a more practical front, I have found that when people focus on limiting added sugars, they limit a bulk of the other junk and ultra-processed foods in their life.

Tracking added sugars also encourages us to read food labels. For example, U.S. manufacturers must list added sugars separately, making them easy to differentiate. Tracking increases awareness and allows for better-informed choices.

A real light-bulb moment for a number of people is when they realize just how many products have added sugars, and products where you might not expect to find them. We all expect that when we indulge in a typical dessert like a bowl of ice cream that we are consuming added sugars. But sugar is now everywhere including but not limited to protein bars, yogurt, replacement drinks, supplements, cereals, granola, sauces, and dressings. It is even added to potato chips.

I recommend staying under thirty-five grams. This is because many people are not eating 2000 calories. It also takes the AHA's (American Heart Association) more stringent recommendations into account.

What's the difference between added and natural sugars?

This is a question asked all the time in the No Excuses Group and a common area of confusion. To put it simply, added sugars are just that, sugar (which has many names) added as an ingredient by manufacturers or after the fact by us.

However, some foods contain natural sugars, which are sugars that are naturally present in the food, and which include the lactose found in milk/dairy products and the fructose found in fruit.

The consensus is that natural sugars are not a problem, mostly because they not only occur in small and diluted amounts, but they also occur in a whole food. In short, packaging matters. Natural sugars, when consumed as part of a healthy diet, do not cause the negative effects that concentrated added sugars do.

And as briefly mentioned above, thanks to recent legislation, food companies selling food in the U.S. need to list added sugars separately on the food label, making it easy to tell the difference.

I'm convinced. But where do I start?

Start by first tracking your consumption of added sugars. This helps you to understand where you are starting. I then recommend setting a realistic goal based on that starting point. Going cold turkey may seem like a good idea, but it often backfires. Once you have awareness and a realistic goal, begin to eliminate those products that are not necessarily important and/or that contribute copious amounts of added sugar to your diet. The key is to get the biggest bang for your buck.

"The best of all medicines is resting and fasting."

BENJAMIN FRANKLIN

If you have not already heard about intermittent fasting, then you have not been paying attention. Yet, even if you have, what intermittent fasting means to you may differ from what it means to someone else. And while I will cover fasting in more depth in a later section of this book, I want briefly to cover it here, as it is a strategy I recommend, especially for women over forty.

In a nutshell, fasting is abstinence from food and drink, and thus intermittent fasting implies periods of non-eating dispersed between periods of eating. Yet, it says nothing about the length of either. For example, when one person says they are intermittent fasting, they may engage in regular prolonged fasts of 24-48 hours, whereas someone else may follow an OMAD (one meal a day) protocol. Still, another daily faster like myself may adopt a regular fourteen-hour extended overnight fast.

I first took a serious interest in fasting after reading a brilliant book that I referenced earlier, *The Circadian Code* by Dr. Satchin Panda.

Panda has spent the past twenty years studying circadian rhythms—natural internal processes that originate within our bodies but that the environment influences. In his book, Panda advocates for a type of intermittent fasting called Time Restricted Eating (TRE).

Panda's research has found that when we eat may be as important as what we eat and how much. His data suggests that restricting our eating window to a minimum of twelve hours has significant health benefits. A fourteen-hour daily fast has even greater benefits, with benefits increasing exponentially as the fasting window goes up.

Both short-term fasts like those implied with TRE and longer fasts such as OMAD (one meal a day) and ADF (alternate day fasting which is a practice of eating one day followed by a day of fasting) have benefits with longer fasts potentially yielding bigger payoffs but also harboring greater risks.

Additionally, research to date suggests that longer fasts are more difficult to sustain over the long haul. Remember, input equals output. If you lose weight via a fasting protocol, be prepared to maintain that protocol for the rest of your life.

I advocate for increasing the fasting window to a minimum of twelve hours and up to eighteen hours.

Increasing the overnight fast can help to restore insulin sensitivity. It may also improve gut health, as it gives your body adequate time to do essential maintenance on the gastrointestinal tract. Likewise, regular fasting windows and mealtimes support the body's natural rhythms. People also report that the hard stop to eating associated with closing their window helps to eliminate nighttime snacking, a prevalent type of non-hungry eating that packs on the pounds. Most importantly, increasing the overnight fast to at least twelve and up to eighteen hours appears to be very sustainable.

There are additional benefits to longer fasting periods, such as those seen with OMAD and ADF. These benefits include better blood sugar control and an increase in autophagy—a process by which the body removes dead and injured cells.

Unfortunately, there are also greater risks such as dehydration, fainting, headache, and electrolyte imbalances. And for diabetics, or anyone taking insulin, it can lead to dangerous dips and spikes in blood sugar. Additionally, the research to date suggests that a lifestyle that involves longer-term fasts is hard to sustain. And sustainability is a critical ingredient when it comes to success.

Finally, athletes and those actively trying to build muscle

may find that fasting, even for shorter periods, can impair performance and decrease muscle gains. At this time, more research is needed to understand the benefits and drawbacks of fasting in this group.[10]

As you will repeatedly hear me say, there is no absolute one-size-fits-all. There are strategies and consequences, both positive and negative, of those strategies and even different consequences for different people.

Benefits of increasing the overnight fast or TRE (shorter duration fasts)

1. Improved insulin sensitivity
2. Improved gut health
3. Increased ability to shed pounds or to maintain current weight
4. A hard stop to eating which can decrease or eliminate non-hungry, late-night eating
5. Better sleep if you stop eating at least 2 hours before bedtime
6. Supports your body's natural circadian rhythms if you keep eating window and meals to a regular schedule

Benefits of longer duration fasts

1. Improved insulin sensitivity
2. Improved gut health
3. Weight loss
4. Improved awareness of hunger signals
5. Increased autophagy

I'm interested in fasting, so where do I start?

Start where you are. Choose an eating window you can adhere to, and then gradually shorten it over time until you reach what I call the sweet spot.

The sweet spot is a point at which you maximize benefits while minimizing costs. This will help ensure long-term compliance.

Fasting is not a weight loss program, though some people are using it that way and achieving short-term success. Of course, most diets do when you adhere to them.

Instead, fasting in all its various forms is a long-term eating strategy that has certain benefits that support our health, which includes reaching and maintaining a healthy weight.

Increasing the overnight fast from twelve to eighteen hours is the one strategy I have seen people succeed with even as they struggle in other areas. What could be easier than eating a balanced dinner at five and then not eating again until breakfast the next morning?

Even morning exercisers can engage in an extended overnight fast without significant consequences.

In the short term, it may take your body a few weeks to adjust to your new eating schedule and why it is best to start gradually. But eventually, your body adjusts.

Non-hungry, boredom, and habitual eating can be tough habits to break. You may find that the desire to eat after closing your window is strong, at least initially. For me, I found a cup of caffeine-free tea or even a piece of sugar-free gum was enough to get me through the craving. Eventually, the cravings subsided.

Of course, like any strategy, you may have to tweak it to accommodate your lifestyle. And if it is not for you, then maybe it is not for you.

This book is not about imposing rules. It is about providing you with strategies that not only work in the short term but are also highly sustainable in the long term.

Beware, though. Despite the benefits of fasting, it has become a fad. A buzzword. Fasting has increasingly become just another way to diet and to restrict calories to lose weight, which is disappointing since it has health benefits that go beyond weight loss and weight maintenance.

What should I eat during my eating window?

Fasting does not give you permission to eat junk. During your eating window, focus on getting in all your fruits and veggies while limiting your added sugar. Also, focus on eating quality whole and wholesome food most of the time.

What about Keto? People I know who fast also do Keto.

Keto has become another darling of the fad fitness industry, but at its core, it is just another eating strategy with benefits and drawbacks.

In another section of this book, I will cover several popular diets currently out there, including Keto and fasting. For now, note that you can pair fasting with another eating or dietary strategy if the strategy is healthy and sustainable. So, no, you do not need to adopt a ketogenic diet to get the benefits of fasting.

Are there risks to fasting?

It depends. For most people, extending the overnight fast from twelve to eighteen hours, particularly if done in a methodical and gradual way, has minor risks. The exception might be those taking meds that require food at certain intervals and those on insulin.

In fact, anyone with a preexisting health condition should discuss any dietary changes with their doctor, and this absolutely includes fasting. Just be sure that when you approach your doctor about fasting, you make it clear what protocol you plan to follow. You may also have to educate them on the benefits.

Longer fasts, while yielding more impressive results, often come with more risk. Potentially serious risk and not just for those with preexisting conditions, either. Again, be sure to do your research and talk with your personal doctor.

Be smart and be practical. Fasting is not a panacea. It is a strategy with benefits and drawbacks that is only as good as your ability to implement it consistently. You can lose weight while fasting, but you can also gain it back.

"Fortify yourself with moderation, for this is an impregnable fortress."

EPICTETUS

Moderation in all things. We are all familiar with this saying. Most of us believe it. Some of us successfully practice it. And we can all think of examples where it is untrue. But when making healthy food choices in a world in which we find temptation on every corner, it is the best way to have the proverbial cake and occasionally eat it, too.

The merits of moderation are many, but the most significant relates to sustainability. Seneca said that everything that exceeds the bounds of moderation has an unstable foundation.

Truth bomb!

Extremes are hard to sustain, especially when we must balance so many things. Our jobs. Our families. Our physical health. Our mental health. Our checkbooks.

And finding a healthy balance when it comes to healthy food can be especially challenging when you consider that too many of us live in an environment that is often at odds with our physiology.

Our bodies have evolved to survive in harsh and unpredictable conditions. We have also developed internal strategies to maintain the status quo in a world vastly different from the one we live in now: a modern world where cheap, ultra-processed, and engineered convenience foods are the rule and not the exception.

In short, we are living in a toxic food environment that does not support health.

Take processed foods. Manufacturers, driven by profit margins and not what is in the consumer's best interests, spend obscene amounts of money researching, developing, marketing, and promoting food that is everything we want (cheap, fast, and tasty) but also everything we do not need (calorie dense, nutrient-void, pseudo foods made from cheap ingredients and designed to have long shelf lives even if they shorten our lives).

In his popular book, *Salt, Sugar, and Fat,* Michael Moss reveals tactics used by the food industry to not only engineer irresistible foods but then to sell them to us by exploiting our psychological weaknesses. Tactics such as fMRIs (functional MRIs), which look at how our brains respond to various foods. Focus groups to understand how to make their product more appealing. Research targeted at increasing sales by figuring out how to sell us things that we might not need and that are not good for us.

The result? Food that tastes good but that is not good for our health and super-sized meals that pad our waistlines as it pads their bottom lines.

Their sole responsibility is to make their investors' money. Keeping us healthy is not a priority. And that is what they do, by giving us what we want instead of what we need.

They not only give us what we crave, but they also do it in such a way that pits us against our natural physiology.

For example, throughout much of human existence, finding a steady supply of calories has been a challenge. It is no wonder we evolved with physiological mechanisms that favor weight gain and not weight loss. Take leptin. Leptin is a hormone produced by our adipose tissue that signals to our body when we are fat enough. Adequate fat stores trigger an increase in circulating leptin, which triggers an area in the brain that affects hunger and satiety.

We know through research that leptin-deficient individuals will not only be obese but will also become obsessed with food and eating. Despite having adequate fat stores (aka stored calories), their brain is not getting the message, so they stay hungry and continue to eat.

Unfortunately, while our bodies have evolved with a robust response to too little leptin by increasing hunger and food intake, it appears less responsive to too much, making it better at preserving fat than shedding it.

As we gain weight, we pump out more leptin. This increasing leptin does not initiate as potent a response as too little. Over time, we may even become leptin resistant, meaning we are even less responsive to too much of the hormone.

When we decide to shed the fat via calorie deficits, two things happen. Ghrelin, leptin's counterpart, increases, causing an increase in hunger. As we lose fat, leptin levels also decrease, which can cause a slew of metabolic responses that favor weight gain or discourage further weight loss.

From a purely evolutionary standpoint, a powerful response to too little fat, which outperforms the response to too much fat, makes complete sense. Our ancestors' biggest threat was not too many calories, but too few.

Today's modern food system has changed that. Calorie-dense food is available everywhere. Moderation is not just about willpower. As far as our body is concerned, it is about survival, which until only recently looked like too little adipose versus too much.

But I don't understand. The theme of this chapter is moderation. Only it sounds like you are saying that moderation is impossible.

Not exactly. Unfortunately, moderating food is not simply a mental construct. What, when, and how much we eat is influenced by powerful biological feedback loops. The brain has evolved to keep us adequately fat. Only what that looks like has changed thanks to a rapidly changing food environment.

In short, moderation can be tougher than it sounds, particularly with respect to the foods we eat and when we eat them.

Moderation also has psychological implications. I want you to help me with a brief experiment. I want you to not think about an ice cream sundae. Okay, go. Do not think about an ice cream sundae.

How did it go?

Exactly. The more you try not to think about the sundae, the more you think about it.

Okay, let's keep going. What is your favorite dessert? Do you notice anything at all? For example, does just thinking about your favorite dessert make you want it?

Now, I want you NOT to think about that dessert.

How did it go?

Exactly. Telling you to not think about your favorite dessert guarantees you will think about it. And thinking about it can often produce a desire to eat it, even when you are not hungry.

This is because there are a number of cues that signal hunger, both physiological and psychological, and that drive us to eat.

So, what's your point?

Moderation is less about eating a smaller piece of pie, and more about learning how to moderate food intake in an environment that is at odds with our physiology. Food is no longer scarce or merely a source of calories. It has personal, emotional, and cultural contexts. And this unhealthy food environment is not always something you can shield yourself from.

Moderation is not only hard; it can sometimes feel impossible!

It is why most diets do not work. They rarely teach people how to moderate food choices over the long haul, which means dealing with an unnatural and toxic food environment. They also ignore the physiological and psychological fail-safes in place to keep us from starving. Instead, they blame any adherence issues on lack of will power and inadequate motivation.

Think about it. If moderation is hard, long-term abstinence is damn near impossible for many of us. And that is exactly what diets tell us to do. Abstain. Restrict. Avoid. They focus on creating calorie deficits, not on building long-term eating strategies that embrace moderation meaningfully.

If only.

And again, all this is interesting, but what's your point?

Regarding eating, moderation can be tougher than it sounds, but still a worthwhile endeavor.

Moderation might resemble:

1. Eating whole healthy foods most of the time (at least 80 percent)
2. Making room for occasional guilt-free indulgences
3. Avoiding overly restrictive dietary strategies
4. Focusing on progress, not perfection
5. Understanding that the cards, or the food, is stacked against us, and that moderation may be harder than we think

"Every human being is the author of his or her own health or disease."

BUDDHIST SAYING

Though a health journey is often inspired by a desire to lose weight, shedding excess pounds is just one advantage to a healthy lifestyle that includes regular exercise. For example, exercise, or rather sustained movement as part of a healthy way of living, provides documented and substantial benefits to every body system from the heart to the lungs to the musculoskeletal system to the brain. If there is such a thing as a magic pill, exercise is most definitely it.

But all too often, people reduce exercise to a means to create a calorie deficit, especially when weight loss is a goal.

I see this all the time. The sweat fest mentality. The idea that if it does not hurt, it cannot help.

Unfortunately, it often does hurt and not just in the way we intend. In my almost three decades as a physical therapist, I have seen too many people seriously injure themselves after embarking on a fitness journey. And this is sad because nothing will sabotage your efforts more quickly than an injured back, knee, shoulder, or limb.

Ironically, exercise alone is not a good strategy for weight loss. Not that it does not help, just not in the way we think.

Thanks to the calories in versus calories out model of weight loss, we have reduced shedding pounds to a simple equation. But as we have already discussed, the body is not a closed system, and the calories in versus calories out model of weight gain and weight loss represents an oversimplification.

Yet, it is using this oversimplified logic that we seek methods to increase our calorie expenditure, believing if we just sweat enough, those pounds will simply melt away.

Only according to research, this is not how it works.

As I pointed out earlier, the body wants to maintain the status quo. It is smarter than we think and has evolved with several mechanisms to preserve our precious fat stores and even get them back if we lose them.

For example, research has shown that an increase in energy expenditure through exercise may be compensated for by expending less non-exercise energy throughout the rest of the day.[11]

Sweat fests also increase hunger, prompting us to eat, often more than what we burned.

Additionally, repeated bouts of calorie-consuming, high-intensity exercise can lead to surges in the stress hormone cortisol as well as an increase in the potential for injury.

While some physical stress is good, too much can be detrimental, especially when we are not paying attention to nutrition, sleep, training methods, and recovery.

You cannot beat your body into shape, though this is exactly the approach many people take.

Not that higher-intensity exercise is bad, just that it is a strategy that is often misused and abused.

It is also not always necessary. In fact, women often lose weight after cutting back on their sweat fests.

Yes. You heard me right. Sometimes more is not better, it is just more.

I want to take a moment to tell you a story about a woman I will call Sue. Sue is a busy mother of three. I met her through a local gym. Sue was without question a badass. She oozed dedication. She worked hard. She tried to eat well. Bought all the expensive protein powders. Counted her macros. Signed up for the fitness challenges. Yet, Sue still struggled with about thirty extra pounds.

What fascinated me about Sue was that she was like so many other women I knew. Women who were struggling to lose weight despite their serious and admirable efforts both in the gym and the kitchen.

Sue also struggled with intense sugar cravings. I got the feeling that when she was good, she was very good, but when she was bad, she could be very bad.

Her grueling workout habits were undoubtedly a big part of the problem. I mentioned this to her. Introduced the concept of cortisol and its effects on the body. She listened but was not ready to hear, at least not yet.

Several months later, she shared a picture of herself on social media in which she had lost quite a bit of weight. In a later conversation, she told me how she had shown up to the gym as always, feeling beaten down. Broken even. In fact, she was so physically exhausted, she had almost face-planted during the CrossFit-style class.

She had finally had enough. She thanked the instructor and walked out, canceling her membership when she got home.

Something had obviously clicked.

She then proceeded to just walk five miles a day, something she often did along with her gym workouts. She also, in her words, stopped treating her body like a trash can. An incredible cook, she applied her talents to creating healthy whole-food dishes. She focused on quality. And within a few months, she had dropped almost thirty pounds.

She has since returned to the gym but is careful to listen to her body. She understands fitness is something you do to maintain the machine, not as retribution for something you ate. She continues to focus on her nutrition, which is a game changer for sure because she realizes you cannot out-train a poor diet.

The moral of Sue's story is that more is not necessarily better. More for her meant working against her body rather than with it. Prior to backing off, her body was always in a state of physical stress. The last thing it wanted to do was to release its fat stores. All that physical stress was also increasing her cortisol levels and contributing to her cravings for high-fat, high-sugar, high-calorie foods. Yet, by easing up on the sweat and instead focusing on quality nutrition, her body got a vastly different message. Not only were things okay, but they were also good. Exceptionally good. So good that letting go of that extra fat was natural. A healthy body seeks to maintain a healthy weight.

And yes. I can already hear the skeptics and naysayers. But before you pass judgment, understand I am not poo-pooing exercise, in general, or sweat fests, specifically. Not even close. What I am trying to convince you of is that sometimes we need to challenge our attitudes about exercise.

Exercise should be about maintaining the body in good working order. Fitness in all areas is best achieved by starting where you are, with an appreciation for all your aches and pains and your present ability and level of fitness.

An effective exercise strategy will challenge you a little but will also meet you where you are currently instead of where you think you should be.

An effective exercise program/movement strategy should also reflect your goals.

Burpees are not for everyone. Running is not for everyone. Deep squats are not for everyone. Two-hour daily workouts are not for everyone. And they are not necessarily necessary, thank goodness.

Exercise (aka regular movement that challenges your body) is about promoting fitness. And when we talk about fitness, we are talking about cardiovascular fitness, muscular fitness (strength and muscular endurance), joint mobility and flexibility, as well as coordination and balance.

A well-rounded exercise program will focus on building all the areas just mentioned with respect for where an individual is starting. Burpees are not appropriate or necessary for everyone or even anyone. Interestingly, in my thirty years of fitness, it is rare to see someone who does a burpee with the correct form. In most cases, when I see people doing burpees, I see an injury waiting to happen and a future patient.

Now, I'm not picking on the burpee. The burpee is not the problem. It is the way most of us use it, or rather misuse it, that is problematic.

Interestingly, it takes only thirty minutes of low-to-moderate intensity activity a day to lower our risk of chronic diseases. And they do not even need to be consecutive minutes. Ten minutes three times a day is just as effective.

If fitness is your goal, sixty minutes of moderate intensity exercise four to five times a week can do the trick. Riding a bike at about 10-15 mph and a brisk walk or a jog are examples. Or depending on your fitness level and time constraints, you might substitute in a few 30-minute HIIT (high-intensity interval training) workouts for good measure.

If performance is your goal, then you are looking at sixty to ninety minutes of moderate to higher intensity exercise six to seven days a week, if not more. And for the record, although performance demands fitness, it does not always promote health. Athletes often push their bodies to extremes that while amazing are not, by default, healthy.

What does all this mean? How much should I exercise and what should I do?

The short answer is *it depends.*

The long answer is *it depends.*

Ideally, you should start where you are.

You will hear me say this repeatedly because it is such an important concept. I might also add to know where you are going. Having a clear idea of your destination is also important.

For example, if you are an overweight fifty-two-year-old, postmenopausal woman with a history of a torn meniscus in your knee who has not been exercising for the last ten years and whose goal is to drop some pounds and improve overall health, the way you approach exercise and movement may differ from a slightly overweight, thirty-year-old female who wants to drop a few pounds, get leaner and fitter, and who has no major underlying conditions and has also been exercising some, though sporadically.

The first woman described may start in the health category. She may need to just focus on lower intensity, shorter duration activities. She will also have to modify exercises based on her limitations.

The second woman may push a little harder from day one with higher intensity, longer duration, and greater frequency workouts.

Both women are starting at different levels because of different physical abilities and limitations. They also have slightly different goals. And while we have not discussed this, they likely have different resources.

Resources can be something tangible, like money for a trainer or access to a gym. Or they might be less tangible, like support from a family member or a more disciplined disposition.

Like I always tell my clients/patients, we all have our crosses to bear, and they are ours and ours alone. You can either figure out how to carry them, unload them or lean on them, which translates to staying stuck where you are.

You choose.

That's great. But you still have not told me what to do.

Bingo. I have not. And to be honest, I cannot. Not in a book, at least. The thing is it really depends.

I can tell you how to improve cardiovascular fitness. I can explain the physiology of getting stronger. I can point you towards exercises that enhance mobility and flexibility. I can tell you that you need to start where you are. I can impress upon you the importance of also knowing where you are going. I can preach the benefits of a comprehensive, well-rounded fitness program, but what I cannot do is prescribe you a program sight unseen.

Okay. But really? What am I supposed to do?

Since I know this is important, I will do my best.

1. Move daily in ways that feel good but that also challenge you a little. And this movement does not have to take place in a gym.
2. Start slow and be cautious. You can always increase the intensity and time tomorrow, but an injury can set you back weeks or even months.
3. Understand your limitations, physical, emotional, and psychological. Know your strengths and weaknesses and have a plan that builds on itself incrementally and methodically.
4. Realize, like every other health promoting behavior, showing up consistently is key. This means building a habit of regular movement through practice.
5. Remember, some movement is always better than none. Maybe every workout is not social media worthy. Just do something. It will help to establish and nurture the habit of moving.
6. Think about your goals. What is your endgame, and how can you support it through a sustainable motion that respects your body at every age and every stage?
7. Think about the big picture. Where does movement fit into your life not just for a few weeks or a few months, but over the long haul?
8. Stop reducing exercise to a means to burn calories, and instead view it to fine-tune and maintain the machine. Ask yourself, does my fitness/movement program make me feel good? Does it increase my energy? Does it lower my stress? Does it help with my back pain? Does it result in better sleep and lower stress levels? Does it support my health and wellness goals?
9. Remember that when it comes to getting leaner, nutrition is far, far more important.

In the accountability group I used to run, I encouraged participants to have a mileage goal where one mile on foot equaled one mile and fifteen minutes of other exercise like biking, swimming, dancing, yoga, resistance training, and really any movement that challenged their current fitness as a one-mile equivalent.

The idea was to choose a goal that was doable, ramping up as needed to support their desired outcome through a sustainable movement program.

Trying to do too much too soon almost never ends well. Remember, you are not embarking on a race that can be won, only run. This is a forever journey, so think about a long-term strategy for movement that feels good.

And do not underestimate the power of simple movements like walking. The National Weight Control Registry is an ongoing research project that started back in 1994. To take part in the study, you must have lost thirty pounds and kept it off for more than a year. Participants complete regular questionnaires to help researchers better understand not only how the participants lost weight but also how they kept it off.[12]

Approximately 90 percent of participants report exercising on average about one hour per day, and walking is one of the most popular forms of movement.

Unless you want to run a marathon, you do not have to train for a marathon.

In my fifties, I am training for life, so I choose activities that support my ability to stay active, sleep well, move without pain, and just enjoy a long and disease-free, quality life. I also choose activities that challenge my strengths and respect my weaknesses. My 50-plus-year-old body, even though well cared for, differs from my 20-year-old body. And that's okay.

Later in this book, we will explore some current fitness trends and why they may or may not be a great strategy for you.

"A good laugh and a long sleep are the best cures in a doctor's book."

IRISH PROVERB

In the private coaching group I used to run, one behavior we practiced was sleep. And we practiced sleep because the connection between sleep, health, and weight is becoming blatantly more obvious as we better understand the function of sleep and the consequences of not getting enough.

For example, too little sleep increases cortisol levels while increasing insulin resistance. Both chronically elevated levels of the stress hormone cortisol and a decrease in insulin sensitivity can contribute to weight gain and an increased risk of many lifestyle diseases.

Studies have shown that a single bad night of sleep can rev up our appetite, particularly for high-fat, high-sugar, calorie-dense foods. It is also associated with the build up of amyloid plaques, which have been indicated in the onset of Alzheimer's.

Lack of sleep may also make it harder to resist unhealthy foods as it can affect our willpower reserve.

Most experts now believe sleep is important not just for maintaining optimal health but for reaching and maintaining a healthy weight.

The question then becomes *how much is enough*?

Things get a little murkier here. Similar to nutrition needs, sleep requirements may depend on life demands, health, age, and medical status.

The general recommendation for adults is an average of seven to nine hours of quality sleep per night. Quality sleep can also be difficult to pin down. Just lying in bed with your eyes closed may not be enough to reap the benefits of a good night's sleep.

It is also possible that you may need more sleep than I do. And the sleep you require on any night may also vary.

A more prudent approach to sleep might be to assess how you feel during waking hours. Do you awake feeling sluggish? Do you nod off during the day? Are you frequently sick? Do you remain sore for days after a workout? Do you find it difficult to concentrate during the day? Do you crave sweets and high-calorie foods? Are you easily stressed?

Answering yes to any of these questions may be a sign that you are not getting enough vitamin Z, as in your nightly zzzzz's.

As we continue to learn more, sleep recommendations may change. For example, there is evidence that deep meditation may offer the same benefits as a solid night's slumber, but in a fraction of the time.

And, as is often the case, learning how to listen to your body and respond appropriately may be the key. Good might not be ideal but it might be good enough.

This is an area where we are learning more every day, but like other lifestyle factors, it is hard to tease out the effects of too little sleep and/or inadequate sleep from the effects of other behaviors.

If you are interested in learning more about sleep, I would highly recommend Arianna Huffington's book, *The Sleep Revolution*.

"The pursuit of perfection often impedes improvement."

GEORGE WILL

Striving for excellence is an admirable pursuit. As Vince Lombardi once said, "Perfection is not attainable, but if we chase perfection, we can catch excellence."

This might be true if you are trying to win a baseball pennant. But my experience is that when building better habits, chasing perfection is not only overrated and unnecessary, but it can also be detrimental.

In fact, chasing perfection is likely to end in failure rather than excellence.

The men Lombardi was speaking to had already built impressive habits through regular practice and repetition. They had mastered the basics of their sport.

Unfortunately, a number of people are floundering as the struggle with even the basics of building a lean, strong, and healthy body.

The problem with chasing perfection is that when we fail, and we will, we often equate that failure to a lack of self-worth or a personal shortcoming. And this often sabotages our efforts to make positive change, a change that is not only hard but takes much longer than we think it should.

If you want to build a lean, strong, and healthy body, focusing on progress no matter how small or seemingly insignificant—not perfection—seems to be the ticket to success.

Lifestyle change really is the act of putting one foot in front of the other, every day, no matter how short the step. The reality is we are not only trying to build new habits, but we are trying to replace old ones.

I see more journeys permanently derailed by chasing perfection than I can count. Not only is perfection not attainable, but chasing it is usually unsustainable. And I hope you are realizing how crucial sustainability is.

Progress, while often light years away from our idea of perfection, implies a step forward. And despite what we think, moving forward is not the result of enormous leaps and bounds, but often the cumulative result of repeated small steps toward our desired destination.

The devil really is in the details, those tiny little everyday details. Our decision to eat an additional fruit or veggie with every meal. Finding a little extra time in our day to get up and move. Turning off Netflix an hour earlier to get that extra vitamin Z.

Making change requires that we start where we are, use what we have, and do what we can.

Being too rigid, trying to do too much too soon, or setting the bar too high are common mistakes.

Instead, position yourself for success by setting realistic goals. Like it or not, lasting change often looks more like the turtle than the hare.

So, where do I start?

Earlier in this chapter, I covered some basic strategies in depth.

1. Eat 7-8 servings of fruits and veggies every day
2. Limit added sugars to under 35 grams a day
3. Increase the overnight fast to a minimum of 12 hours
4. Eat whole healthy foods at least 80 percent of the time
5. Learn how to indulge guilt-free
6. Move on most days in ways that feel good and challenge your body a little in some way
7. Implement a comprehensive fitness program that addresses all areas of fitness to include cardiovascular fitness, muscular fitness (strength and endurance),

mobility, flexibility, balance, and coordination.

8. Get 7-8 hours of quality sleep on most nights

This represents an ideal or, at least, an admirable goal. But that does not mean it is where you start. Remember, you start where you are. If you are currently barely eating two to three servings of fruits and veggies a day, a more realistic short-term goal might be to up your intake to three to four servings. Then, once you are consistently mastering three to four, you can move the goalpost a little and start shooting for four to five.

Regarding the overnight fast, if late-night eating is a big problem, you might start with an overnight fast of ten or eleven hours and then methodically and incrementally increase.

Currently a sugarholic, you might simply first address sugar by tracking it. This will build awareness. Then you can slowly limit the amount of added sugar you consume based on your ground zero.

Exercise is no different. You need to consider your current habits regarding exercise or lack thereof and your current fitness level and move forward from there.

And yes, it will take time, more time than most people want. But whether we want to accept this or not, mastering the behaviors that support our ideal really is the only way to reach and stay at that ideal.

Everything else is a quick fix or a temporary one.

Let me repeat that. Everything else is a quick fix or a temporary one.

How much change and how quickly we can make it will depend on us. Our starting point, our resources, our level of motivation and determination, our commitments, our support structure, our current health status, and our level of fitness. Even our personality can be a relevant factor.

In that respect, I cannot tell you how long it will take, only that it is usually much longer than we desire. I can also tell you that setting yourself up for success (focusing on progress) rather than overshooting (chasing perfection) will increase your chances of succeeding even if not on your desired timeline.

Perfection is unrealistic, and pursuing perfection can lead to a level of fatigue that will often prompt us to not only throw in the towel but to throw it away. A focus on progress, no matter how small, is a better strategy Those tiny wins not only add up, but they also help to build the consistency and habits to keep us where we want to be.

Bottom line: strive for regular progress, not perfection.

"Success does not come from what you do occasionally. It comes from what you do consistently."

MARIE FORLEO

If there is one lesson I hope you garner from this book, it is that you are what you repeatedly do. Not what you say you will do. Not what you want to do. Not what you plan to do. But what you do do. On any day or at any given moment.

Every thought you have which manifests in every action you take is a vote for some version of yourself.

It is that simple.

Want to write a book? Some talent is helpful, but unless you show up to write the book and put your thoughts down on paper, it does not get written.

Want to become a doctor, nurse, lawyer, firefighter, physical therapist, or accountant?

You must show up. You must check the boxes. And you must act in a way that is consistent with achieving those end results.

And if you want a lean, strong, and healthy body, you must act in ways that support a lean, strong, and healthy body.

And if you want a lean, strong, and healthy body that lasts longer than a hiccup, you must consistently and repeatedly act in ways that support a lean, strong, and healthy body.

SUCCESS - HOW YOU DO IT VS WHAT YOU DO

A s I mentioned before, building a lean, strong, and healthy body is as much an art as a science. And to drive home this point, I want to tell you another story. My three sons play baseball. My oldest pitched. As a physical therapist with a strong background in kinesiology, I became fascinated by the mechanics of pitching. So, doing what I always do when I want to learn more about a topic, I bought a few books.

One book I bought called *The Art and Science of Pitching* was written by Dr. Tom House. House started off as a pitcher and eventually founded the National Pitching Association. He spent a sizable chunk of his post-pitching career studying the mechanics of pitching. And thanks to modern technology that allows us to put markers on a pitcher and slow down and analyze the video, we now know more about the mechanics of an effective pitcher than we once did.

Interestingly, he also used this technology to study not just today's greats but also well-known pitchers from the past. And while every pitcher had his own unique style that appeared quite different, a closer examination showed that they shared key similarities. Through his research, House identified several key traits that all successful pitchers possessed. The idea is it is their shared attributes, as opposed to their differences, that made them successful.

And that is what I want to do now here for you. Having been at this a long time, I have had the opportunity to not only educate myself and study the various relevant topics, but I've also spent decades observing other people, some of them wildly successful at building and maintaining a lean, strong, and healthy body.

Popular diets and fads focus on what these people do differently, but I am convinced it is what they do the same that makes the difference.

What follows is my best assessment of the similarities in their approaches.

"When you have clarity of intention, the universe conspires with you to make it happen."

FABIENNE FREDRICKSON

Intention

All the wildly successful people I know live life with intention. Their decisions are based on choice and not by chance. Their success is not an accident. It results from an intention that includes specific behaviors that support their goals, whatever those goals might be.

They might not all employ the same diet or exercise strategy, but they have one, and it is usually a well thought out approach they have put time and effort into developing and implementing.

Intention can manifest itself differently. In a broader sense, intention can offer clarity which helps you shape your long-term goals and your long-term strategy to achieve them. But on a more basic level, intention describes those things you plan to do on a regular, if not daily, basis.

For example, I want a lean, strong, and healthy body. I know the things I need to do to make that desire a reality. But unless I have a clear intention, the gap between desire and reality is often too wide to bridge.

So, every day I set a clear intention. I plan on eating seven to eight servings of fruits and veggies. I plan to fast for fourteen hours by closing my eating window at 5 p.m. I plan to limit my added sugar to under thirty-five grams. I plan to eat mostly whole, minimally processed foods. I plan to move in ways that challenge my body, and I plan to sleep at least seven hours.

My intentions are crystal clear. And even if I cannot always check every box every day, having clear intentions increases the chance that I will check any.

Intentions provide a checklist of sorts that becomes the basis for the decisions we make throughout the day. It is the framework from which we function in our daily lives, and which can move us toward some desired outcome. Most notably, every successful person I know lives a life filled with intention.

Rarely do we succeed at anything by mistake or accident.

Intention means having a plan, a clearly defined set of behaviors and actions that support our goals. But it might also mean having a backup plan or Plan B. A good Plan B allows us to stay true to our intent, even on our worst days.

My intent on most days is a fourteen-hour fast that starts at 5 p.m. and lasts until 7 a.m. But if life prevents me from doing this, and I end up eating after my window normally closes, my plan is to delay my first meal the next day to help make up the difference.

And remember, a Plan B does not have to be comparable. In fact, it might look different and instead be a modified intention.

For example, if my plan were to take a yoga class after work, but something comes up and I cannot, Plan B might be to spend at least ten minutes at home moving instead. Here, the type of movement and/or the duration is not as important as following through on my intention.

Not only is something always better than nothing, the act of showing up, even if it means modifying your original intention, has power.

If reaching your goal represents a blossoming flower, then intention represents the seed.

"We become what we want to be by consistently being what we want to become each day."

RICHARD SCOTT

Consistency

Building on my flower analogy from the previous section, if intention is the seed, then consistency is most definitely the water. Need proof? Look at anyone you know who has succeeded at anything. While they may have employed different strategies, I guarantee most of them employed their strategy consistently.

You can drive, walk, crawl, bike, run, sprint, or jog up the mountain. The mode you use to get there may vary, but you will not get there unless you continue to move forward.

Again, you are not what you say you will do. You are not even what you intend to do. You are what you consistently do.

In Angela Duckworth's best-selling book, *Grit*, she writes, "Enthusiasm is common. Endurance is rare."

In my three decades in the health and wellness industry, I have seen people start a health journey. They are excited. They are determined. They have finally grown tired of their own excuses. They are ready to act. Ready to finally make that change. They buy the latest diet book. They purchase a new gym membership. They join a fitness challenge. Maybe they even join my No Excuses Facebook group. And they are all in until they are not. Enthusiasm is great, but it will not get you very far.

When I look at people who maintain lean, strong, and healthy bodies over the long haul, it is not necessarily the grand gestures that make the difference. It is the repeated, daily ones that matter most. Their routines. Their habits.

They understand that consistency is key.

And consistency can be tricky. It means being able to pace yourself. Overcome by enthusiasm and impatience, many people embrace unrealistic and unsustainable methods. They want results, and they want them now. I often hear people claim they are going to do a more extreme program until they lose weight, then they will focus on making a more sustainable change.

Only that rarely, if ever, works. Almost never.

Consistency requires that we be honest with ourselves about where we are starting and what resources we have available. It also means being patient and acknowledging that real change takes time. Though long-term strategies rarely produce the quick and dramatic results we desire, they result in the long-term change we hope to obtain.

So, whatever your ultimate strategy, you need to keep in mind that your ability to employ that strategy consistently may be more important than the strategy itself.

"I accumulated small but consistent habits that ultimately led to results that were unimaginable when I started."

JAMES CLEAR

Habit

Habit is the child of intention and consistency.

The successful people I know come in all flavors. They are not necessarily more talented or less handicapped. They get tired. Their motivation wanes. Life throws them a gazillion curve balls, too. They are real people with their own unique baggage.

The biggest difference is unlike those who are struggling, they have formed habits that support their goals. So, when they find themselves caught in one of life's inevitable storms (and they have them, too) their autopilot (aka habits) takes the wheel.

Consistency is without a doubt the key to forming better habits, and habits are the key to making lasting sustainable change.

Again, I would encourage you to think of someone you know who has succeeded at anything (wellness-wise or otherwise), and you will see that in most cases they have adopted habits that support their desired outcomes.

Habits are the stones that pave the road to success. Without habits, we must depend on motivation or enthusiasm in the moment, neither of which is dependable or up to the task.

But if we want to make sustainable long-term change that not only serves us during the highs but carries us through the lows then habits reign supreme.

"The key is not to prioritize what's on your schedule, but to schedule your priorities."

Priorities

One of my favorite sayings is *if it is important to you, you will find a way. If not, you will find an excuse.*

We often pay lip service to some ideal. We say we want something, but when it comes time to pay the proverbial piper, we sometimes have a million excuses. And this is usually because the perceived cost of a particular behavior in the moment outweighs the perceived benefit.

People who succeed at making choices that support their long-term goals are often much better at prioritizing their time. They understand the deep and meaningful *why* behind their goals, and they really want that thing which they say they want because they have tied it to their values. They do not just want to lose weight. They want to lose weight so that they can spend more quality time playing with their kids. They not only want to be healthy and fitter because they value health and fitness but also because they understand the implications their health and fitness has on their ability to show up in their daily life as the best version of themselves.

They do not find the time. They make it.

If you constantly make excuses, it is very possible you lack a commitment to whatever it is you think you want. And maybe it is because you lack clarity about what it is that you really want and why. Or maybe you have failed to tie it to your personal values (those things you say matter to you.)

All of us make choices. And not all choices that support our goals feel good at the moment we make them. But we make them because we realize that they are essential to achieving whatever it is we hope to accomplish. And that is why we need our priorities straight. We need to understand and appreciate the long-term value (to us) of what we are doing and accept that sometimes the right thing is the hard thing.

Successful people are often experts at delaying gratification because they understand their priorities and they appreciate the value of what it is they are trying to accomplish. They have made the connection between certain behaviors and how those behaviors relate to those things that are important to them.

If you are struggling to implement a new behavior, it is worthwhile to do an internal audit and re-evaluate what you want and then make sure your priorities reflect and support that thing you say you want.

"Success is stumbling from failure to failure with no loss of enthusiasm."

WINSTON CHURCHILL

Persistence

Jim Watkins said, "A river cuts through rock, not because of its power but because of its persistence."

Persistence is consistency on steroids. It is the ability to stay focused on our goals and true to the process, even when faced with the unpleasant sting of failure.

Persistence does not attach our effort to some arbitrary metric for success. Instead, it means showing up on the good days and the bad days in equal measure and pushing forward even in the absence of perceived gains.

Persistent people do not get distracted or discouraged by failure.

They understand that failure is inevitable. It is not a matter of *if* but of *when*. There will be days and weeks where they will do all the right things, yet they will not reap the rewards for their efforts. Forward progress is rarely a straight line. It is a series of steps forward and steps backward.

But they also are not distracted by success. They realize that just as failure is not fatal, success is not final. They stay focused on the process and not the outcome because they know that the outcome at any moment is temporary and a reflection of the process.

Too often, we face a setback or even a success, only to be derailed. Faced with failure, we get discouraged. Faced with success, we get complacent.

Long-standing success requires persistence at all stages. This idea that we reach our goal, usually a weight goal, and then live happily ever after is as much a problem as allowing temporary setbacks to defeat us.

Those successful at building and maintaining a lean, strong, and healthy body continue to engage in the process. Day in and day out. They play what I call the long game. And they never stop playing.

"Real transformation requires real honesty. If you want to move forward, get real with yourself."

BRYANT MCGILL

Honesty

Being successful at building the body of our dreams often requires honesty. We pay lip service to some ideal. We imagine ourselves in the abstract. In this ultimate vision of ourselves, we may be super fit, we may be stunningly beautiful, we might even be wildly successful.

But saying we want something and being willing to invest the time, energy, and effort it takes to get it are two completely different things.

People struggle because they lack commitment to what it is they say they want, or they do not truly believe they can ever have it. Another possibility is they make the process harder than it need be, almost guaranteeing that it is harder. Whatever the case, they almost never get it.

They are lying to themselves.

Instead of acknowledging the disconnect between what they claim to want and what they will do for it, they make excuses, which are just another form of self-deceit.

The most successful people I know are honest with themselves, not only about what they want, but what it will take to get there. And they are not afraid to call out their own bullshit. They understand excuses do not produce results.

They are not afraid to challenge the process or their attitudes about the process when it is not working. And they rarely delude themselves about what it will take to not only claim but also keep the prize.

Being honest with ourselves about what we want, what it

will take, what we will do for it, what we can realistically do for it, and why we might not follow through with it are all hallmarks of the brutal, yet nonjudgmental honesty most successful people possess.

If you are not getting what you want, you may be lying to yourself without even realizing it. You may be deceiving yourself about what it is you truly desire. You may lack an understanding of what it will take to get it. You may be kidding yourself about what you will do for it not just in the best of times but also in the worst of times. Understanding the true cost of achieving a goal is essential. And being willing to pay the price is non-negotiable. It is not simply enough to want something. We need to be able and willing to do the things necessary to support the outcome we desire. That takes honesty.

"Acknowledging the good that you already have in your life is the foundation for all abundance."

ECKHART TOLLE

Gratitude

At the risk of sounding preachy, it has been my experience that those who want more and eventually get it are often masters at first appreciating what they already have in the moment. And this is especially true of my super fit and healthy friends and colleagues.

A grateful spirit allows them to approach their goals with a sense of abundance rather than one of scarcity.

It also provides them a much-needed perspective as they work toward something bigger and better while allowing them to do so thoughtfully and mindfully because their happiness and inner contentment is not contingent upon the success of some arbitrary goal but a manifestation of it.

They seem intuitively to understand that appreciating what you have is one of the best foundations for building something you want.

When pursuing any goal, failure is inevitable. As we have already discussed, it is not a matter of *if* you will fail but rather of *when*. And it just so happens that gratitude for what you already have is one of the most sturdy and dependable bridges between where you are and where you want to be. Without it, failure can feel like a big, dark, bottomless hole that sucks you down into the abyss. Yet with it, failure is just another pothole in the road, inconvenient but not impassable.

Gratitude takes the pressure off such that it fosters patience, forgiveness, and compassion with yourself and a process that is necessary to accomplish anything of value.

And there you have it: seven traits shared by people who not only build a lean, strong, and healthy body but also maintain it.

Intent
Consistency
Habit
Priorities
Persistence
Honesty
Gratitude

The rest is often negotiable. What we eat, when we eat, and how we eat may be quite different. The same is true with exercise.

I have shared my personal approach, which is based on the science currently available, my understanding of it, my education, my observations working with others, and my own personal experiences.

But there are many strategies that can help build a lean, strong, and healthy body if you address intent, consistency, habit, priorities, persistence, honesty, and gratitude.

If you are struggling to build and maintain a lean, strong, and healthy body ask yourself if you possess and apply the previously mentioned qualities. Do you live with intent? Do you consistently show up? Have you had success forming habits that support your goals? Do you understand your priorities? Are you persistent in the face of failure and success? Are you brutally honest with yourself about what you want, what it will take, and what you are realistically willing to do for it? And do you have a spirit of gratitude regardless of where you are?

Depending on your answers, your chosen mode of transportation up the mountain (aka diet or exercise plan) may not matter because even if you get started and have short-

term success, you may find that you cannot keep going and
sustain and support that success.

FINDING YOUR STRATEGY

I wanted to summarize the previous section of this book before moving on.

To this point, we have focused primarily on the idea and importance of having a process and all the things that might derail, impede, or sabotage that process.

Things like unrealistic expectations or timelines. Destructive or counterproductive mindsets. Ineffective or flawed strategies and inconsistent implementation, the pitfalls of seeking perfection over progress, and the limitations of motivation.

We also outlined the importance of intent, consistency, habit, priorities, persistence, honesty, and gratitude as they relate to reaching our goals regardless of the strategy.

I offered my general guidelines/formula for building a lean, strong, and healthy body, a template that is based on my experiences, and described exactly what that might look like (eating fruits and veggies, limiting sugar, increasing the overnight fast, etcetera).

I also tried to impress upon you that sometimes how you do something may be as important, if not more, than what you do.

In the second half of this book, I want to explore several popular nutrition, exercise, health, and lifestyle topics in greater detail, with the end goal of not only helping you find a strategy that supports a lean, strong, and healthy body but a personalized strategy that works for you and works long term. I purposely cover questions and topics that come up repeatedly in my No Excuses Facebook group because they are areas where many people struggle. I also make a point of covering the body and body systems as they relate to health as opposed to just weight loss while emphasizing the difference between the two.

I have tried to present the information logically, though, at times, I had no choice but to digress. I encourage you to read this section with an open mind and curiosity, understanding that finding a strategy that works for you in both the short and the long term is as much an art as a science.

Emotional and Non-Hungry Eating

It is no secret that we often eat and overeat for reasons that go well beyond biological hunger. We are bored. Maybe we are tired or stressed. Maybe we are enticed by the food that is in front of us. Unfortunately, the availability and convenience of high-calorie, high-fat food has made it all too easy to overindulge, eating to the point where it can negatively impact our waistline and our health. It is also why emotional and non-hungry eating is a topic that comes up frequently in my No Excuses Facebook group. It is a real problem.

Non-hungry eating refers to eating for reasons other than hunger. For example, eating out of boredom or habit are common examples of non-hungry eating. **Emotional eating** is a type of non-hungry eating that we will address separately because of its prevalence and complexity. It results when individuals use food (or liquid calories) to cope with emotions.

What causes non-hungry eating?

Boredom, habit, and/or access to food are often the driving force behind mindless non-hungry eating. External cues drive our desire to eat. Polishing off a bucket of popcorn at the movie theater. Devouring a hotdog and cotton candy at the ballpark. Binging on an entire bag of potato chips while binge-watching Netflix. Does any of this sound familiar?

With non-hungry eating, there is usually a trigger. A visual cue. A smell. A ritual that has forever paired a food or eating behavior with a specific activity, such as pumpkin pie on Thanksgiving and birthday cake on our birthday. It could also be driven by the taste of food and/or how that food rewards the brain.

Habit influences boredom/habitual eating, and habits are powerful things. They are the brain's attempts to conserve valuable and limited resources. Our ability to switch to autopilot is essential for functioning in a complex world. We would be overwhelmed without this automatic mode.

Unfortunately, for too many of us, our habits (or automatic mode) sabotage our health goals and do not serve our best long-term interests.

What about emotional eating?

Did you know that *stressed* spelled backward is *desserts*? Coincidence? Probably. But we can all relate to the craving for certain comfort foods when we have had a rough day or are dealing with difficult emotions.

Emotional eating is a type of non-hungry eating that goes beyond boredom or habit. Food becomes a coping mechanism. We eat to deal with an emotion. Sadness, anger, frustration, fear. These emotions make us uncomfortable, so we stuff our faces to blunt that emotion and feel better, even if only temporarily.

Unfortunately, many of the foods we choose to self-medicate are calorie-dense, nutrient-void, and high in fat and sugar. Even worse, the relief we get by indulging in our comfort foods is often transient and can leave us feeling worse in the end. Ironically, like drugs and alcohol, fat and sugar have addictive qualities. This is likely because once upon a time they were in limited supply or extremely desirable in a food environment where calories were harder to come by and starving to death was a real possibility. And while eating a couple of cookies (at least on the surface) is less harmful than taking drugs, in its most severe form, emotional eating can lead to binge eating (eating the whole bag of cookies and maybe more), a serious eating disorder that often goes well beyond food.

In my experience, emotional eating is more of a problem for women than men, though men are certainly not immune. There are several explanations for this difference between the sexes. For example, traditionally a woman might be more likely to shop for and prepare food, making her relationship with food more complex. A woman also experiences monthly fluctuations in powerful hormones that contribute to cravings for fatty and sugary foods. Hormonal shifts associated with pre-menopause and menopause often come into play. Women are also the fatter sex because our bodies were designed to not only provide calories for ourselves but also for our offspring. Finally, although this is changing, the objectification of women's bodies has historically placed pressure on them to meet an unrealistic standard of beauty which can further contribute to an unhealthy relationship with both their bodies and food.

Emotional eating also has a physiological basis. As we already mentioned, once upon a time, the threats we faced did not just feel like life and death, they were life and death. As a result, when under stress—physical or emotional—our body releases hormones like cortisol and adrenaline. Cortisol can have a profound impact on not only hunger but also the foods we choose to satisfy that hunger. During times of stress, we crave fatty, sugary, high-calorie foods. Our distant ancestors had limited access to both sugar and fat. We also had to work harder for our calories back then, unlike today when calorie-dense processed foods surround us.

Elevated cortisol levels can also impact the quality and quantity of our sleep, which further increases cortisol levels. Disrupted sleep in turn affects leptin and ghrelin, two important hormones that regulate hunger and satiety. And both stress and lack of sleep can impact insulin sensitivity.

It is a vicious cycle.

Strategies to Deal with Emotional and Non-hungry Eating

When it comes to non-hungry eating, whether boredom/habitual eating or emotional eating, the first step to getting it under control is to acknowledge that it is a problem and to recognize that it is not just a mental battle. Non-hungry eating, and especially emotional eating, has a biological basis, and biology is a powerful driver of our behavior. Giving into a craving does not make you a bad or a weak person. It makes you human.

It is also important to understand that willpower is a limited commodity. We often blame a lack of willpower when we cave to a craving, yet most experts agree that willpower is a finite resource. And while some individuals have a bigger reserve than others, most of us will reach the bottom of the barrel at some point. When you accept the limitations of willpower and motivation, you will appreciate the importance of planning to ensure better eating practices.

Mindfulness is Key

Habit drives boredom and habitual eating. Therefore, you must address your habits if you hope to get non-hungry eating under control. This starts with mindfulness, the ability to be aware in the moment and to make conscious choices rather than simply react. This is easier said than done since habits, by definition, are the brain's attempt to bypass a mindful state. The point of autopilot is so that you do not have to waste time or energy thinking about a particular task. What this means is the brain will resist your efforts to change, at least initially.

The only way to change a habit is to stop yourself and take an inventory of your motivations and your choices. *I want a cookie.* Okay, are you hungry, tired, or bored? Do you want the cookie simply because it is there, and it smells and/or looks good? Does the benefit of eating that cookie (the enjoyment you experience at the moment) outweigh the costs (gaining weight)?

Sometimes the answer may be *yes*, and that is okay. The point of mindfulness is to make a conscious decision rather than an automatic one. And it takes practice. Lots and lots of practice.

Overcoming emotional eating also requires mindfulness. Emotions like anger, fear, frustration, and sadness are normal. Generated unconsciously, emotions are automatic, and we have no control over the emotions we feel in the moment. What we do have control over is how we deal with those emotions once they manifest. Again, it is not always what happens to us that matters as much as how we react.

We avoid emotional discomfort at all costs. So, when sad, we eat or drink to make ourselves feel better. When angry, we throw things, scream, and/or down a gallon of butter pecan to calm the angry beast within. When afraid, we seek comfort through binge-watching Netflix and binge-eating pasta. Obviously, eating to soothe ourselves is not necessarily always a bad thing. Coping mechanisms serve a purpose even if they can have unwanted side effects. Sadly, however, for too many of us, the consequences of emotional eating are worse than the emotional stressor we are trying to cope with. In short, the cure (what makes us feel better at the moment) is sometimes worse than the disease (our discomfort).

We need to learn how to be comfortable with being uncomfortable.

A mindful approach to eating allows us to create distance between ourselves and the emotion or the impulse at the moment.

I am angry. Huh. Okay. I do not like how that feels.

By creating distance and allowing yourself to experience the emotion non-judgmentally, you give the emotion a chance to play out. Most emotions peak and then wane. The point is to let the emotion(s) pass without reacting.

Mindfulness requires awareness, and building awareness takes practice. It is a skill like any other we must master, or at least improve with time. And it starts with your head with the story you tell yourself. With the inner dialogue you create and with your attitudes about food, about eating, and about yourself.

Real-life strategies for overcoming non-hungry and emotional eating

Overcoming non-hungry and emotional eating can be hard. It takes practice and consistency to replace old unproductive behaviors with new, more productive ones. It also requires some clear intention, which is why in the following section I have provided several specific and practical strategies to help you deal with non-hungry and emotional eating.

1. Acknowledge that all forms of non-hungry eating (including emotional eating) are not only normal but also have a biological basis

You are normal. You are not weak. You are not even excessively flawed. You are human, and you are not alone. Non-hungry eating is not a personal shortcoming or a moral failing. In fact, much of it is driven by a body that is well adapted for food scarcity but not for food plenty. Today's food environment is at odds with the feedback systems that have evolved to keep us healthy and safe.

2. Understand the limitations of willpower

We all have a limited supply at our disposal. Knowing our limits is key. Because once we understand and embrace our personal limits, we can plan accordingly.

What things drain you? When is your willpower reserve likely to be low? Do you have trigger foods? What specific actions can you adopt so that making healthy food choices is easy, not just during the best of times but also during the worst of times?

Knowing the answers to these questions will allow you to

devise a mindful approach toward eating. For example, if you must buy chips for another person in your household and chips are a trigger food, keep them out of sight or make them harder to reach. Research has shown that simply making a food physically less accessible is a viable deterrent. Along the same lines, if making bad choices after a long day at work is a problem, meal planning or having a quick, healthy food option available in a pinch can be the difference between eating a gallon of Rocky Road and something a little more nourishing. When you are tired, it is unlikely you are going to have the energy or motivation to cook or prepare something healthy. Not when it is so much easier to reach for the chips, a bag of cookies, or other quick, unhealthy, readymade food option.

3. *Stop and think before you put it in your mouth*

Whether we are talking about habitual/boredom eating or emotional eating, the ability to pause in the moment and contemplate what we are doing and why we are doing it is critical. Initially, this is hard. It takes energy and effort. Our brains (which are lazy) will resist. They have evolved to conserve energy and resources for more important matters. But do not worry. Though it will take conscious time and effort in the beginning, it will get easier as you adopt new habits and learn new and better strategies for dealing with stress and emotions.

4. *Create distance between you and the impulse or emotion*

Angry and reaching for *Ben and Jerry's*? Set a timer. Go for a walk. Take a bath. Drink a cup of tea. Write your emotions/ motivation in a journal. If you can create space between yourself and the impulse or emotion, it will often pass. And you can even give yourself permission to eat whatever it is you were going to eat after a specified "cooling down" period. Whatever decision you make will result from a conscious choice rather than prompted by a knee-jerk reaction.

5. *Learn positive ways to deal with stress*

Coping strategies are important. Learning to deal with stress in a healthy way is the goal. Meditation, yoga, exercise, reading, relaxation, a hot bath, a cup of tea, aroma therapy, journaling, traditional therapy, a massage, and getting adequate quality sleep are all positive ways to deal with stress. The key is to find a more productive method to process our negative or uncomfortable emotions. Again, this takes awareness, mindfulness, and practice. Lots and lots of practice. Yet, over time, you will rewire your brain, and instead of turning to food for temporary comfort, you will utilize these other more productive strategies.

6. *Be kind to yourself, always*

Kenny Rogers was onto something with his lyrics from *The Gambler.* "You've got to know when to hold'em. Know when to fold'em. Know when to walk away. Know when to run." Sometimes giving in to a craving is the best thing we can do. Why? Because sometimes that craving serves a purpose. We have all tried to resist a craving for something we really wanted, not because we were hungry, but because we wanted it. Instead, we ended up eating ten other things we did not want, only to end up eating what we really wanted anyway. Food is not just about eating calories. And sometimes the benefits of eating that cookie outweigh the costs. Sometimes it is better to eat the cookie, satisfy the craving, and then move on. Not everything you put in your mouth need qualify as a health food or address hunger. By allowing yourself these indulgences, you minimize the unproductive and often toxic effects of guilt. Along the same lines, do not strive for perfection. Sometimes good enough is good enough.

7. *Focus on nourishing your body, not punishing it*

Food is beautiful. It tastes good. We need it to survive. It has a cultural and emotional context. Eating is an enjoyable experience.

Our food choices often reflect our complex relationship with food which is further complicated by an unnatural food environment where food is not only available 24/7, but also easy to get, convenient, and cheap. Food companies have engineered food that is inexpensive, fast, and irresistible. Then they market it aggressively, exploiting our weaknesses to increase their profits. But that is the world we live in. And to honor your health, you need to make mindful choices. This has never been more difficult. Fortunately, it gets easier, especially if you can harness the power of habit to work for you rather than against you. It takes effort. It takes time. There are forces conspiring against you. In the end, your ability to love yourself and make decisions that honor your health because you love yourself is critical. Choose foods that nourish. Stop seeing healthy eating as punishment or penance. Instead, understand that the foods you eat are a way to care for and nourish this awesome body you live in. Stop using your body as a trashcan and making excuses.

Motivation and Consistency

EVERY. SINGLE. DAY.

That is what it takes. Not dramatic efforts, just consistent ones.

We briefly addressed motivation earlier, but I want to spend more time here because it is another topic that comes up frequently in the No Excuses group.

People want to know how they can find the motivation to do all *the things* they need to do consistently, especially when so many other things are competing for their mental, physical, and emotional resources.

Hopefully, at this point in the book, you realize that building better habits is the best way. The question then becomes *how does one go about building better habits?*

As I mentioned previously, many books cover this very topic. I have referenced one of my favorites, *Atomic Habits* by James Clear. And while I cannot do justice to such a complex process in a few pages, I am going to at least try to outline the basics.

Identify Your Why

When people request to join my No Excuses Facebook group, I ask them *why*. While not everyone tells me, a number do. Some say they want to get fit. Others say they want to get healthy. Many say they want to lose weight, and quite a few say they need help to lose the excuses.

Whatever the case, even if not provided, there is always a reason they ask to join. Unfortunately, these superficial *whys* often miss the mark because they do not get to the real *why*, the deep and meaningful reason behind their desire to get fit, eat better, lose weight, lose their excuses, and/or exercise more.

I am talking about the *why* behind the *why*. Why do you want to get fit? Why do you want to eat better? Why do you want to lose weight? Why do you need to lose the excuses or exercise more?

You might want to get fit and healthy so you can be more involved with your kids or grandkids. Maybe you want to lose weight to feel more confident and comfortable in your own skin and, by default, become a better life partner. Maybe you want to reverse a chronic disease like diabetes, so you will be there for your family for as long as you can.

Whatever your deep and meaningful *why*, it should reflect your core values: those things that you say are important to you. Things like happiness, health, family, integrity, honesty, learning, kindness, relationships, etcetera.

Remember, if it is important to you, you will find a way. If not, you will find an excuse. Identifying your deep and meaningful *why* and relating it to your core values helps to make it important.

Thus, finding time to exercise is not a selfish, negotiable act that takes time away from your family or other life obligations. It is a necessary act and investment in your future to help ensure you will be there for those you care about as long as possible and in the best physical and emotional shape to boot.

Eating better foods is not just about losing weight. It is about leading by example so that your kids or family or friends, too, can reap the benefits of whole, healthy foods.

There on tons of free core value worksheets available on the internet. Once you know your core values, you can then ask yourself how doing *the things* (exercising regularly, eating well, sleeping better, and managing stress) relate to your deep and meaningful *why*, and how that deep and meaningful *why* supports your core values.

If you can do this, if you can connect the dots between the behaviors, your *why*, and your values, all *the things* (moving consistently, making better food choices, prioritizing sleep) become non-negotiable because they support something you value. They are not selfish. They are necessary. They are important, and therefore they should be a priority. And while motivation might be nice, it is unnecessary.

Most people do not get up every morning and go to work just because they love their job and have nothing better to do (some may...but many do not). They do it, at least partly, because they want a paycheck, and they want a paycheck because it allows them to pursue other things they value.

If you can tie your vision to your values, all *the things* become your job. These things simply become what you do because they support you in your efforts to live life meaningfully.

I just cannot help myself; I cannot afford to eat healthy. I do not have time to prepare food, prep/cook. I lack the emotional, physical, or financial resources to do what I need to do.

How often have you made an excuse for making the easy choice? The truth is we absolutely have the resources we need to take care of ourselves. And the harsh reality is we really cannot afford not to. Do not forget, self-care is about giving the world the best of you, instead of what is left of you. When we are completely honest with ourselves, the biggest barrier we sometimes face in making better choices is ourselves. This brings me back to mindset. The only way to control what you put in your mouth is to start with your mind. It all starts between the ears. The best way to get the motivation to exercise is to make the connection between movement and the quality of your life.

Understand the Dichotomy that Is Motivation

We have already discussed how a lack of motivation is a fallacy since we are always motivated to do something.

Unfortunately, our motivation in the moment may not always reflect our long-term goals.

Identifying your *why* and relating it to your core values can certainly help increase your motivation for doing the right things, but there will still be times when the motivation to do what feels good in the moment wins out. And that is because often there are no immediate consequences for doing the thing that feels good as opposed to doing the thing that might not feel good but that supports your desired result. In fact, there is often an immediate reward.

Going back to the job analogy. Staying home from work simply because you want to sleep in is not an option. It might even get you fired. On the other hand, hitting the snooze button rather than getting in your workout or ordering fast food rather than planning out a nutritious meal does not always come with immediate negative consequences. Just the opposite. And that is why it is so easy to make the easy choice that feels good. Sure, there are long-term consequences, but often so far down the metaphorical road, they do not provide enough of a deterrent.

That is why you need intention, consistency, habit, priorities, persistence, honesty, and gratitude: the traits we discussed earlier.

Intention gives you clarity about what it is you need to do. Consistency at practicing checking off the boxes helps to build habits. Getting your priorities straight ups the ante. Persistence keeps you from surrendering to failure, which is inevitable, or success, which is temporary. Honesty ensures you will call out your own bullshit when you try to make excuses for not honoring those things you say you value. And gratitude offers you a much-needed perspective that allows for failure even as it lays a foundation for success.

Motivation in the moment is nice but certainly not a requirement. Commitment to your desired outcome is.

Have a Plan

It has been my experience that those who have the most success with building and maintaining a lean, strong, and healthy body not only have a strategy, but they also have a plan, and not just any plan, a specific checklist of sorts that focuses on sustainable behaviors that support their desired end game.

And please, please, please do not overlook or underestimate the importance of sustainability when formulating your plan. If you do, failure is likely. You must not only do all the things for a few weeks, a few months, or even a year. You must continue to do *the things* forever and ever, amen. Again, most people know they need to make a lifestyle change, yet when they embark on their journey, they have chosen a path so hard, so unsustainable, there is very little chance they will achieve anything that even remotely resembles long-term success.

Without a detailed and sustainable plan, you are leaving things up to chance and putting yourself at the mercy of your motivation in the moment. This might not be a bad thing if we were always motivated to do the right thing. So, have a plan, a specific set of behaviors that will support your goal, and make sure those behaviors are achievable and sustainable. You can always up the ante, but only after you have mastered the basics.

Make the Right Choice as Easy and Accessible as Possible

This might seem like a no-brainer, yet we routinely make getting healthy and fit harder than it need be, setting ourselves up for failure before even starting.

News flash! Starving and/or depriving yourself via restrictive diets is not a requirement for losing weight or getting leaner. Neither are 2-hour long daily and intense sweat fests.

Yet, this is the approach many people employ. Then, to add insult to injury, they tie their success to three arbitrary numbers on the scale. Another mistake.

The best approach or strategy is the one that facilitates long-term, lasting, and sustainable change because it supports your goals over the long haul. And it is almost always the slow and steady approach.

This means starting where you are and setting incremental and realistic goals to get you to where you want to be.

It also means figuring out how to make the right choice as convenient as possible. Getting your workout clothes ready the night before. Meal planning or meal prepping so that when life gets hectic, you are prepared. Pairing a new desired behavior with an old established one. Finding a supportive network to provide you with accountability or moral support. These are just a few ways you can set yourself up for success.

Make the Wrong Choice Harder or More Uncomfortable

Just like making the right choice easy and more convenient can facilitate us doing the right thing, making the wrong choice harder or less convenient can deter us from behaviors that do not serve us.

As we have covered, not only does the wrong choice often not result in immediate discomfort or negative consequences, but it often feels good. And this makes doing the right thing even more challenging.

Making the wrong choice less attractive or associated with more immediate pain is a valid strategy to increase motivation in favor of the desired behaviors.

For example, making junk food less accessible by not buying it or keeping it out of sight or physically harder to get to increases the immediate cost of that food, and thus it can be an effective deterrent. Having a workout partner that depends on you to show up is another way to make the wrong choice more costly. It is one thing to hit snooze when you are only letting yourself down. It is a completely different thing to let down a friend.

Commit to the Plan

Do not give yourself an out. I repeat. Do not give yourself an out. Your plan is a contract with yourself. This does not mean you have to beat yourself up if you do not always follow through. And remember, that is what your Plan B is for. As we have already discussed, striving for perfection often sets us up for failure. But I am not talking about perfection. I am talking about commitment, intention, and a sincere effort to follow through with your plan not only on your best days but also on your worst days.

And if you have set good goals (aka SMART goals) this should not be too difficult.

In case you are unfamiliar with the term SMART goal, it is an acronym that delineates several characteristics of an effective goal.

S stands for **specific**. For instance, eating better might be a way to express your overall goal, but it is not specific enough to be instructive. Eating three servings of fruits and three servings of vegetables each day is much more precise. And conveniently, it also doubles as not only your intention but also a specific plan/checklist.

M stands for **measurable**. A good goal is measurable. For example, not only is the previous example of eating three fruits and three veggies each day specific, but it is also measurable. You either eat that many servings or you do not.

A stands for **achievable**, which simply means that even if challenging, there is an extremely high probability with some effort that you can realistically reach your goal. And this is so important because setting a goal you cannot meet sets you up for disappointment, no matter how nice it sounds on paper or no matter how noble your intentions.

R stands for **relevant**. A SMART goal should support your desired outcome. If running a marathon is your ultimate long-term goal, a SMART short-term goal could be any short-term or daily goal that helps you to achieve your primary long-term goal.

T refers to **time-bound**. A goal (whether large or small) needs to be connected to a time frame to be effective, otherwise it is just hanging out there all by itself with no clear parameters. In the fruit and veggie example, the goal is time-bound by the twenty-four hours in a day.

A **SMART** goal can be long-term or short-term. And you will have both. For example, your SMART long-term goal might be to run the NYC Marathon in six months. It is specific. It is measurable. It should be achievable. It may be relevant to your bucket list, and it is time-bound. A SMART short-term goal might specify a daily or weekly training goal, such as running three miles every other day. In short, most long-term goals will require short-term goals as well. If it is a big goal, it might even require several tiers of goals from big to small.

Daily goals really are just intentions that provide you with a detailed plan.

Getting fit is an ideal. The behaviors that get you to that ideal are the goals.

Seek External Support

Securing a supportive network can be an invaluable source of motivation, inspiration, and accountability. It is what my No Excuses group is all about.

Finding a workout buddy, joining a support group, and investing in a trainer or a group fitness class are all examples of how you can find support on your journey.

As we discussed previously, it is one thing to hit snooze when you are the only person you are letting down. But it is a whole other situation when you are letting someone else down.

Likewise, surrounding yourself with others who have similar goals and/or already having success with behaviors you want to adopt can be extremely motivating thanks to the effects of peer pressure, which cannot only be negative but also positive.

In their book *Connected: The Surprising Power of Our Social Networks and How They Shape Our Lives*, Dr. Nickolas Christakis and Dr. James Fowler show just how powerful the company we keep can be, even when it comes to health behaviors and outcomes. According to their research, we exert an influence of three degrees over friends, our friend's friends, and our friend's friend's friends. What this means is that not only does our immediate circle influence our behavior, but it also has a ripple effect that reaches far beyond our own personal interactions.

Hang out with people who drink beer and eat pizza on Friday nights, and you are more likely to do the same as are your friends and their friends. Hang out with people who work out regularly and eat healthy and the influence is just as strong.

In summary, if you want to be a writer, hang out with other writers. Want to complete a triathlon? Befriend others who are already competing. Want to engage regularly in healthy behaviors? Surround yourself with those who are not only trying but who have been successful.

Think Outside the Box

Sometimes the biggest barrier we face on a health and wellness journey is our way of thinking about the process.

We have fixed ideas not only about what it takes but about how it needs to be done. This often causes us to see barriers rather than opportunities when faced with limited resources.

For example, a lack of time is one of the biggest obstacles people face when trying to get more active. It is not necessarily that they do not want to exercise or even that they hate to exercise. It is just that figuring out how to fit in those movement sessions amidst life's other pressing demands seems impossible. Lack of time is such a common excuse that researcher and author Martin Gibala dedicated an entire book to identifying just how long it takes to get in an effective workout. His findings, which he shares in *The One Minute Workout,* might surprise you. To better understand the benefits of steady-state cardio and shorter length HIIT (High-Intensity Interval Training) protocols, his team used muscle biopsies to study cellular adaptations. His results suggest that it really does not take all that long to get the benefits of exercise if you are strategic in your approach. In fact, his *one-minute workout*, a ten-minute session that includes one minute of very high-intensity movement, is not only effective at improving cardiorespiratory fitness (as effective as a 60-minute steady state session at a moderate intensity), but it also burned just as many calories thanks to the effects of EPOC (Excess Post-Exercise Energy Consumption). In short, lack of time is not a valid excuse for not exercising.

Thinking outside the box, or at least our box, can significantly boost our chances of being successful.

CALORIES, MACROS, AND SCALES

To count or not to count. That is another topic that comes up frequently in my No Excuses Facebook group.

The obsession members have with counting calories, usually to create a calorie deficit, demonstrates just how popular and ingrained the calories in versus calories out model of weight loss and weight gain is.

If only it were that simple.

The fitness and diet industry are mostly to blame for this oversimplification as fitness gurus continue to push the calorie deficit approach to weight loss. Yet, we have already briefly discussed why calorie deficits, which often work in the short term, do not work so well in the long term. Proponents of the calorie deficit model of weight loss assume the body is a closed system. They neglect the fact that our bodies have evolved to protect our precious fat stores at all costs, and prolonged calorie deficits not only send the body into a defensive mode (slowing down our metabolism), but they also trigger an offensive mode (increasing hunger and cravings). And this is a big part of the reason they are unsustainable.

But more importantly, the calorie-deficit model of weight loss often does nothing to address the underlying reasons we ate more than we needed to begin with. Being healthy is the default state of our body. If it were not, we would never have made it this far.

A more comprehensive approach is to ask ourselves, *what went wrong? Why is there extra weight to lose? Why did we overeat in the first place?*

Is it our relationship with food? Is it physiological and psychological hunger gone wrong? Is it too little movement, lack of sleep, or stress? Are our hormones out of whack? Do we have stomach issues? Is it the poor quality of calories we are consuming? Is it merely the sheer number of calories we are consuming? Are we metabolically sick? Have we developed unhealthy habits around food and movement?

Simply tracking calories and/or limiting calories does little to address the underlying problem(s). In a well-functioning healthy body, at least in theory, calories should take care of themselves.

Look around. What other animal in the wild struggles with obesity?

Why is that?

Certainly, our unnatural food environment, characterized by calorie-dense, nutrient-void, easily accessible food is a factor, but it goes much deeper than that.

Set Point Theory

Set Point Theory is a popular and even widely accepted theory that challenges the conventional wisdom of the calories in versus calories out, calorie deficit model of weight gain and weight loss.

According to Set Point Theory, certain areas in the brain function as a thermostat of sorts that carefully monitors our weight, and which can cause several biological, physiological, and hormonal fluctuations designed to maintain the status quo (in this case, our weight) and often despite and in contradiction to the calories in versus calories out model.

Imagine a thermostat that is set to a temperature range.

If the temperature drops too low, the heat kicks on. If the temperature gets too high, the air kicks on. This is the type of system believed responsible for keeping our weight stable within a set or predetermined range. And it makes complete sense from an evolutionary and survival standpoint. A body that has the flexibility to adapt well to a variety of conditions while maintaining homeostasis is really in our best interests.

According to the theory, weight is not just a function of the calories we take in, but rather of our set point.

The key to losing weight then is not necessarily a calorie deficit, but instead changing our setpoint. Only, how we do that is not exactly clear. It is important to understand that our set point may be more of a set range than one specific point. This range is likely dictated by internal factors like genetics and hormonal health as well as external factors such as the type, amount, and frequency of the calories we eat. Exercise, sleep habits, and stress likely play a role as well.

Certain proponents of the Set Point Theory believe that it is important to never lose more than 10 percent of your body weight at a stretch since losing any more than 10 percent of your body weight triggers all those fail-safes meant to keep our weight within our set point range. For example, losing too much weight too quickly can trigger a slowing of your metabolic rate or BMR and/or a change in the hunger and satiety hormones that drive eating behavior. Restricting weight loss to 10 percent of weight followed by a period of maintenance is believed to allow a natural shift in the set point range, or a resetting of your thermostat.

Others, like Dr. Jason Fung author of books including *The Obesity Code* and *The Diabesity Code*, suggest that the best way to change our set range is by eating better quality calories and eating less often to help prevent large and frequent insulin spikes. Fung argues that too much insulin, not necessarily too many calories, is the real culprit behind weight gain and difficulty losing weight. And though not everyone agrees, he is not alone.

The take-home point is simply that focusing primarily on calorie deficits by restricting calories may not be a great long-term strategy because it does not address the real problem, the set point. Furthermore, Set Point Theory, if accurate, may explain why so many people regain weight.

But what about tracking calories?

Eating too many calories can be a problem even if not the root problem. And for some, tracking calories may be part of the solution, even if not the whole solution. Tracking can raise awareness about consumption and help to reinforce boundaries in a food environment where food cues are mismatched with many of our internal fail safes. Again, too many poor-quality calories were rarely a problem for our ancestors.

Yet, the decision to count calories is personal and has both positive and negative consequences. Tracking calories increases awareness and accountability around food which is a good thing. It can help us to identify proper portion sizes and prompt us to read labels. And in a world where mindless eating has become as much a sport as an art, it may provide us a much-needed hard stop to eating.

On the other hand, many people track calories hoping to create a calorie deficit, and as we have already discussed, whether a set point or range exists, research has shown deficits are not an effective long-term strategy for getting and keeping the body of our dreams. For starters, calorie counting and calorie deficits tell us nothing about the quality of food consumed, which may be just as important as quantity. Calorie counting and calorie deficits also fail to address the underlying issues that contribute to overeating in the first place since hormones and other internal and external cues heavily influence hunger. Finally, calorie counting can become exhausting while calorie deficits are often unsustainable. Both can contribute to unhealthy attitudes about food, ultimately sabotaging our efforts.

Interestingly, the profound psychological consequences of calorie deprivation were best illustrated by the post-World War II Minnesota Starvation Experiment led by Ancel Keys.[13] Conducted in the 1940s, the original purpose of this study was to develop a protocol to deal with starved, undernourished soldiers returning home after the war. Thirty-six males between the ages of twenty-two to thirty-three ate a diet of about 2000-3200 calories for three months. Calories were then reduced to about 1500 calories for the next six months and delivered over two meals per day to approximate the diets of active soldiers. Subjects walked twenty-two miles a week and kept a daily diary. On average, participants lost about 25 percent of their starting weight.

The next twelve-week phase involved a controlled re-feeding period in which subjects received different diets reflecting a variety of macronutrient combinations and supplementation. The last phase of the study included an eight-week unrestricted re-feeding phase in which participants could eat whatever they wanted.

The results of the study served as a basis for creating instructional pamphlets used by aides in Europe and Asia to best address the nutritional status of returning soldiers. Interestingly, the most notable observation made during this study was the impact that the calorie restriction had on both the physical and psychological health of the participants. During the semi-starvation phase, subjects showed several metabolic markers consistent with a decreasing metabolism, including decreased heart rate and body temperature. Likewise, during both the semi-starvation phase and the re-feeding phase, patients became depressed, withdrawn, and obsessed with food. A handful of participants even reported dreaming of food.

Though we cannot extrapolate the findings of this study to all calorie-restricted diets, they offer insight into the potential dangers of prolonged calorie restriction and may help explain the poor long-term outcomes associated with almost all diets that stress calorie restriction as a primary strategy to lose weight.

Finally, it is also worth noting that unless you have gone through some sophisticated testing, nobody really knows how many calories they need or do not need to maintain or lose, so it is kind of a shot in the dark, anyway. And, as observed in the Minnesota Stravation Experiment, the body can and will eventually adapt to fewer calories. What this means is the body simply figures out ways to be more efficient. I do not know about anyone else, but I would like to eat as many calories as possible or as hunger dictates as opposed to an arbitrary amount based on some rough estimate of a rough estimate for somebody else. Why train your body to survive on less if you do not have to?

In conclusion, while calorie deficits yield poor long-term outcomes, the decision to count calories may depend on you, your personality, your goals, and what you find helpful. And it may change. For example, you might find it worthwhile to track calories early on to raise awareness and make better-informed choices about the foods you eat. And maybe you do not. It is up to you. Ask yourself, *is this behavior serving me? Is it helping me to make better choices and establish sustainable habits?* If the answer is *yes*, then go for it and keep going for it for as long as it continues to serve you.

What about macros? I understand why it may be futile to count calories, but don't I need to track my macros?

Once again, the answer is that it depends. For those unfamiliar with the term, *macros* refer to the macronutrients we eat which are carbohydrates, fats, and proteins. We will learn more about these individual macronutrients shortly, but for now, let us stick with the upside and downsides of tracking them.

The idea behind counting macros is that there is an ideal

ratio of each that we should strive for based on our health and fitness goals.

Yet, despite claims to the contrary, we just do not know if an ideal exists and if it does exist what that ratio looks like or if it differs for different people.

There may be a benefit to eating a balance of carbohydrates, protein, and fat at every meal, only what that might realistically mean for an individual could depend on a multitude of factors.

Tracking macros has similar advantages and drawbacks as counting calories. It tells you a little more about the composition of the diet, yet still does not give you any information about the overall quality of food consumed.

If you really want to count something, I recommend starting with servings of fruits and veggies, grams of added sugar, overnight fasting intervals, and hours of quality sleep.

In my experience, when you focus on eating more fruits and veggies (seven to eight servings), limiting added sugars to under thirty-five grams, and observing a minimum twelve-hour fasting window, the calories and the macros often take care of themselves.

The scale lies and a few other things you may already know

Since we are talking about counting and tracking things, it seems like a good time to address the scale and how it fits into the big picture.

Few things hold more power or sway over us than the scale. This is particularly—though not exclusively—true of someone trying to lose weight. But like counting calories or macros, the answer to whether you should weigh yourself is *it depends*.

Earlier in this book, we established why the scale is not a great method for measuring and gauging success, even if our primary goal is to lose weight, or, more accurately stated, get leaner.

That said, tracking weight can be a legitimate source of accountability and motivation for select individuals.

If you choose to weigh yourself, (and honestly, who can resist) I would caution you to keep the scale's limitations in mind. It is also helpful not to fixate on any single reading.

Daily weigh-ins are more likely to cause you unnecessary disappointment and frustration. Instead, if you must track those three little numbers, try weekly or every other week measurements, and, even then, do not get overly invested in any single reading. Instead, trust in the process and look for change over time. Progress often resembles a zigzag as opposed to a straight line.

For those in the maintenance phase, more frequent weighings (at least initially) may be beneficial, as, during this stage, individuals can struggle to find a new balance.

Whatever you decide, keep in mind that the scale only reveals our gravitational pull at a single point in time. If you must use it, use it with an appreciation for its shortcomings.

DEMYSTIFYING MACROS

Macros have become another buzzword/term in the fitness industry. We are told they are important. That if we ever hope to reach our health and wellness goals, we need to count, track, and balance them. But what exactly are macros, and why are they so important?

Macros refer to the three important macronutrients: carbohydrates, protein, and fat. Despite popular rhetoric suggesting otherwise, all macronutrients can and should play a role in a healthy eating strategy as they all help to meet our nutritional needs, not just for calories but also for micronutrients such as vitamins and minerals.

Historically, there has been significant confusion around these macronutrients and how they fit into a healthy eating strategy. In the '80s, fats were demonized, a misguided campaign that led to the copious consumption of highly-refined carbs since manufacturers often replaced the fat they removed with refined sugar. Since then, the pendulum has swung, and now carbs have found themselves on the proverbial chopping block.

The reality is neither fat nor carbs are inherently bad. They are inherently good. Yet, thanks to a food industry that has created pseudo foods that are not only nutritionally inferior, but even unhealthy, and a fitness industry that does not do a good job at conveying nuances, teasing out the good information from the bad presents an ongoing challenge for many.

Given the attention that so many people are giving macros, I could not write a book on health and wellness without addressing these totally essential though often misunderstood dietary components. Once you understand what they are and their unique role in your health, you may better understand what all the noise is about, but more importantly how they all can and all should fit into your personalized nutrition strategy.

Carbohydrates

What are carbohydrates?

Though often maligned, carbohydrates are an important calorie source that when eaten in their natural form provide energy along with a boatload of vitamins, minerals, phytonutrients, and fiber.

Structurally speaking, they are chains of one or more of the monosaccharides glucose, fructose, and galactose.

A **monosaccharide** is a single molecule structure made of a 6-carbon ring in the case of glucose and galactose and a 5-carbon ring in the case of fructose.

A **disaccharide** is a two-molecule structure. There are three disaccharides: sucrose, lactose, and maltose. Sucrose is composed of a molecule of glucose and fructose. Lactose is formed by pairing galactose and glucose, and maltose is formed by combining two glucose.

Fructose and maltose are naturally occurring sugars found in plant foods. Maltose is also an intermediate substrate formed during the digestion of long-chain carbohydrates. And finally, lactose is a naturally occurring sugar found in milk.

Monosaccharides and disaccharides are collectively referred to as **simple sugars** or simple carbs. These naturally occurring simple sugars often provide the sweetness we derive from various intact foods.

Longer chains of glucose, or **starches**, also exist in nature and the foods we eat. Unlike simple carbs, starches contain extended chains of glucose strung together. These longer chain structures are referred to as **complex carbohydrates.**

Both simple and complex carbs contain four calories per gram and can be digested and broken down into their component parts (glucose, fructose, and/or galactose), absorbed, and then used for energy.

Glucose is our body's fuel of choice.

The body accesses the energy stored in glucose either **aerobically** (in the presence of oxygen) or **anaerobically** (in the absence of oxygen).

Glucose is so important that the body has a system to ensure blood levels do not get too high or too low. It also has a system for storing glucose in the muscle and liver as **glycogen** (more immediate energy) or as **adipose** (slower burning energy).

Fiber is another type of carbohydrate found in plants that the body cannot digest. Fiber is further classified as **soluble** and **insoluble** based on its physical properties.

While we cannot digest fiber, the microbes that populate our gastrointestinal tract can. This microbial digestion produces short-chain fatty acids that are essential to our overall health. Likewise, fiber adds bulk to the diet, which not only keeps us feeling full sooner and longer, but also helps to keep us regular. Finally, soluble fiber can reduce the amount of dietary cholesterol absorbed, which lowers LDL (aka bad) cholesterol levels.

It is important to point out that intact foods like fruits, vegetables, whole unrefined grains (such as quinoa and wheat germ), beans, lentils, and legumes not only contain a mix of macronutrients (carbs, protein, and fat), but they also contain a variety of carbohydrates including naturally occurring simple sugars, complex carbs, and fiber.

We label certain foods as carbs. Unfortunately, this can be an oversimplified way of viewing the food since it does not take into consideration all the other macro-, micro-, or phytonutrients also present.

For example, when you eat a piece of fruit or a whole grain like quinoa, you are getting a mix of simple sugars, complex carbs, and soluble and insoluble fiber besides a bunch of micronutrients (essential vitamins and minerals) and phytonutrients (powerful, disease preventing and curing phytochemicals like polyphenols and flavonoids). And with a food like quinoa, you also get protein and even a small amount of fat.

Carbs are not only *not* unhealthy, but they are also packed with nutrition. Of course, we are talking about intact foods/carbs (aka good carbs), or foods in an unprocessed or minimally processed form, as opposed to the highly-processed pseudo foods (aka bad carbs) that comprise an increasingly larger part of our diet. And when talking about all the macronutrients, not just carbohydrates, it is critical to understand the difference because it can literally make all the difference.

To further explore the nuances between good and bad carbs, let us start with corn. In its intact form, corn is an excellent source of all three carbohydrates: simple, complex, and fiber. It also provides several essential vitamins and minerals as well as phytonutrients.

Now take that same ear of corn and chemically treat it to isolate the fructose and glucose. Then further refine it to create a syrup we call high fructose corn syrup. Add that super sweet syrup to highly-refined flour, eggs, milk, etcetera, and you have something that populates our grocery store aisles and that is also vastly different from one of its natural ingredients: corn.

Let us consider another example, a whole intact grain like long grain brown rice. We cook the rice and serve it with stir-fried veggies. The whole grain not only adds complex carbs and fiber to our meal, but it also adds important nutrients like iron and the B-complex vitamins as well as a little protein, a little fat, and a good dose of fiber.

In contrast, remove the nutrient-dense outer two layers of the intact grain's germ, keep the inner pulp, bleach it, and use it to make rice flour that is then combined with the high fructose corn syrup described previously. Again, you end up with one of the many food products on the grocery store shelf. You will also have something vastly different from its intact whole-grain ingredient. It is now something that is not only nutritionally inferior but also something that is not well suited for our bodies.

Carbohydrates from intact foods are not only not bad, but they are nutritional powerhouses that are well suited to a healthy body. Equating them to processed foods made from a refined version of the original natural food is unfair.

When talking about carbohydrates, it is important to understand the difference between nutrient-dense and nutrient-diverse intact foods and processed foods made using those intact foods but only after a refining process that strips away many of the vitamins, minerals, phytonutrients, and fiber, leaving behind a nutritionally inferior product and something that has almost nothing in common with the original food.

Intact foods high in healthy carbohydrates include vegetables, fruits, beans, lentils, legumes, nuts, seeds, whole intact grains, and dairy.

Processed foods that are high in less healthy and even unhealthy refined carbohydrates include any baked product made from refined flour, white or wheat, pasta, white rice, cereal, chips, added sugars, crackers, cookies, candy, ice cream, flavored yogurt, sweetened granola, etcetera.

What about diabetes? Don't carbs cause diabetes?

The answer to this question is not a straightforward *yes* or *no*. And to fully understand the complexity of the relationship between carbs and diabetes, it may be helpful to first lay groundwork for this discussion by exploring diabetes in greater depth.

Firstly, there are two types of diabetes: **type 1 diabetes** and **type 2 diabetes**.

Type 1 Diabetes

Once referred to as juvenile diabetes because it historically occurred early in life, type 1 diabetes is an autoimmune disorder where the body's immune system attacks the pancreas, the organ which makes insulin. As a result, type 1 diabetics are not producing insulin and thus need an artificial source. Left untreated, type 1 diabetes can be deadly.

Insulin is a hormone required to clear glucose from the bloodstream and transport it into the cell where it can be used for energy or stored as either glycogen (quick energy stored in the liver and muscle) or adipose (slower energy stored as fat).

Type 2 Diabetes

Type 2 diabetes, previously called adult-onset diabetes because it used to occur later in life, is a lifestyle disease in individuals that can have an underlying genetic predisposition. What this means is that if you have the gene/epigene, your environment and daily choices can turn it on.

Type 2 diabetics make insulin, but over time their cells develop a resistance to it. As a result, their pancreas pumps out even more insulin. Early in the disease process, type 2 diabetics produce plenty of insulin, but over time the pancreas may peter out. This is the point at which a type 2 diabetic will also need to take artificial insulin.

Though different, both type 1 and type 2 diabetics are metabolically sick since their body is not producing enough insulin or their cells do not recognize it.

Because carbohydrates are repeating chains of glucose, their consumption and digestion cause a spike in blood sugar. How much and how fast the glucose from carbs enters the bloodstream depends on the type of carbohydrate and the amount of carbohydrate and other macronutrients and nutrients ingested in the meal. A healthy body deals quite well with moderate and infrequent glucose spikes. Unfortunately, too many of us eat too many of the wrong things and way too often, which can lead to both frequent and large blood sugar spikes that result in subsequent large and frequent insulin spikes, both of which can eventually contribute to insulin resistance.

Glycemic index is a score given to a food that reflects how quickly the body absorbs the glucose present in that food.

The greater the proportion of complex carbs and fiber to simple carbs, the lower the glycemic index. Also, the less processed the carbohydrates in the food, the slower and more gradual the rise.

Glycemic index has limited application since it only tells us how a certain amount of a particular food can affect blood sugar when eaten in isolation. It does not take typical serving sizes or mixed meals into consideration.

To provide a more meaningful number, experts developed the **glycemic load,** which considers a traditional serving size. It, too, has some limitations but may be a better tool than the glycemic index.[14]

So, while fruits high in natural sugars may have a higher glycemic index, they often have a low glycemic load thanks to their high fiber and low carbohydrate count for a typical serving.

Diabetes experts encourage diabetics to eat a well-rounded, nutrient-diverse diet that includes all intact (natural/whole) foods, even those high in carbohydrates. This is because intact/whole foods provide a ton of health benefits that nourish all body systems. They also provide a mix of carbohydrates, including fiber.

That said, how carbohydrates fit into a diabetic's diet may

vary and depend on the individual, the type of diabetes, where they are in the disease process, and even stress, sleep patterns, and exercise habits. Unfortunately, simply avoiding carbohydrates does nothing to address the underlying problem, at least in type 2 diabetes. High blood sugar is not the problem. It is a symptom. Learning how to eat a whole-foods diet that includes healthy, intact, carbohydrate-rich foods as well as adopting other behaviors such as regular exercise, better sleep habits, and adequate stress management can improve or even reverse type 2 diabetes.

But do too many carbs cause diabetes?

Well, it depends on what one means when they say too many carbs. There is mounting evidence that our increased consumption of highly-refined carbohydrates, which includes added sugars along with the amount and frequency we are eating, contributes to obesity and the increasing incidence of metabolic diseases like type 2 diabetes.

In Dr. Jason Fung's popular book, *The Obesity Code,* he outlines how the insulin resistance characteristic of type 2 diabetes requires two things: large insulin spikes and frequent insulin spikes.

Thanks to our penchant for and the availability of highly-refined foods and the fact that we are not only eating constantly throughout the day but also well into the evening hours, too many of us are creating the environment necessary for insulin resistance and type 2 diabetes to occur. Add in terrible sleep patterns, stressful lives, and inconsistent movement and exercise habits and it is no wonder that type 2 diabetes numbers are surging.

In *Nature Wants Us to Be Fat*, Dr. Richard Johnson claims that the high concentration of fructose in added sugars contributes to the development of metabolic diseases independent of its effect on weight.

In short, carbs do not necessarily cause diabetes, but eating too many processed carbs might be a contributing factor both as it relates to weight gain and obesity but also independent of weight gain and obesity.

Take Home Point:

The carbohydrates we consume via whole intact foods differ from the highly-refined carbohydrates we consume via processed foods. Carbohydrates, as found in nature, are not bad. On the contrary, decades of research tell us they are good. Very good.

On the other hand, the food processing of carbohydrates produces a nutritionally inferior product that is not only *not* good for us but in excessive amounts can be bad for us.

Carbohydrates alone do not cause diabetes. However, lifestyle choices and unhealthy eating patterns, including diets high in refined carbs, especially added simple sugars, likely do.

Protein

If carbohydrates are the most demonized macronutrient of this decade, protein is the most overrated. This is not to imply that protein is not important. If you learn anything from this chapter on macronutrients, I hope you learn that all macronutrients are important.

But just as the excessive criticism of carbohydrates is undeserved, so is our uncanny obsession with protein and eating more.

What is protein?

Found in the foods we eat, protein is a complex molecule or macronutrient formed by a group of building blocks called amino acids. These amino acids, once digested and absorbed, can then be used to build necessary proteins like muscle, skin, organ tissue, and enzymes, or other nitrogen-containing substances our body needs to function, such as DNA and RNA. Like carbohydrates, protein also contains four calories per gram, which the body can use for energy, especially in the absence of sufficient carbs.

There are twenty amino acids. Nine of these are essential, which means our bodies cannot make them, and they must come from the diet.

Proteins are further classified as complete and incomplete. A **complete protein** provides all twenty amino acids, including the nine essential amino acids. An **incomplete protein** provides amino acids, but not all twenty.

Animal proteins are complete (or high-quality) proteins because they provide the full range of amino acids needed for good health, while most plant proteins do not and thus are incomplete proteins. Two exceptions would be soy and quinoa, which are complete plant proteins.

Complementary proteins are two or more incomplete plant proteins eaten together, like beans and rice, that alone do not provide all the amino acids we need but when eaten together they do.

Proteins like carbohydrates are digested and broken down into their component parts (in the case of protein - amino acids, dipeptides, or tripeptides) before they are absorbed and transported to the liver. The liver, which regulates levels of amino acids in the blood, can then use these dietary amino acids to make the amino acids our body needs for building its own proteins or shipped off to other cells to be used by those cells.

If you eat more protein than your body needs, the amino acids will undergo deamination, which requires the removal of the nitrogen-containing amine group from its carbon skeleton, rendering it in a form that we burn for energy or store as fat for later use. (Yes, the body stores excess protein as fat.) The cleaved amine group, which is toxic to the body, is removed via the formation of urea.

It is also worth noting that our body recycles amino acids. So, when a body protein like muscle breaks down, those amino acids go into an amino acid pool—figurative and not literal—where they are reused if needed.

The recommended protein intake varies from source to source and often depends on age, activity level, fitness/performance goals, and overall nutritional status, including carb consumption. For example, carbohydrate is protein sparing. What this means is that if you are not eating sufficient carbohydrates to meet your energy needs, protein may be used for energy instead of being spared for the purpose of building tissue.

Likewise, those engaging in intense training or experiencing an active growth spurt may require more protein to account for an increase in anabolic processes.

Most people can get more than sufficient protein without trying. This is because protein, both complete and incomplete, is well distributed throughout the foods we eat. All intact whole foods, including most plant foods, provide protein.

The frenzied push for eating more protein is less a reflection of our needs and more a talking point for fitness gurus who are always looking for something to sell us. And protein bars, protein supplements, protein powders, and protein shakes are perfect profit generators because they often have substantial mark-ups and profit margins.

Ironically, though we generally consume more than sufficient protein to meet our needs without trying, less than 10 percent of us eat the recommended amount of fiber.

We are so busy filling up on our processed protein powders that we do not have room for all those nutrient-laden plants, that not only provide a significant source of protein but also fiber. Nuts, beans, lentils, legumes, and whole intact grains are not only great sources of complementary plant proteins, but they also contain fiber that feeds and promotes a healthy gut microbiome.

The USDA recommends that 10-35 percent of our calories come from a mix of animal and plant protein sources. For someone eating 2000 calories a day, 20 percent would equate to about 100 grams of protein per day.[15]

While this might sound unattainable, it really is not, especially if you are eating a whole-foods diet.

But I'm an athlete. Don't I need to eat more protein?

Not necessarily. Athletes are eating more calories overall, so they will also eat more protein by default if they are eating quality whole foods most of the time. While there are always exceptions, we do not have to work all that hard to meet our protein requirements, again if we are eating quality foods most of the time. And if we are not eating quality foods most of the time, we have bigger problems than not getting enough protein.

What about protein supplements?

Whenever possible, nutrition should come from real food,

and this includes protein. Many supplements touted as excellent protein sources are in fact heavily processed, pseudo foods that are loaded with artificial sweeteners, colors, and other questionable ingredients.

They are also unnecessary. Our bodies evolved to eat real foods, and processed foods, whether carbs, proteins, or fats, seem to be equally bad for us. Interestingly, supplements, including most protein powders, are highly processed food products. Ironically, the same people who are quick to bash processed carbs and refined oils often don't hesitate to consume processed, hydrolyzed protein in the form of protein powders.

The best way to meet your protein needs is to eat a diet with a good mix of plant proteins from whole food sources with animal proteins (dairy, eggs, fish, and meat) to a lesser extent.

Can I eat too much protein?

As previously mentioned, excessive protein eaten beyond our amino acid needs is used as energy or stored as fat. This process requires deamination and produces a toxic substance we must excrete via urine.

For those of us with healthy kidneys, this is unlikely to be a problem. However, if you have kidney disease, it could be detrimental.

Additionally, there is mounting evidence that diets high in animal protein may increase our risk for certain cancers, partly because they are not so great for our gut microbiome. However, there is still much we do not know. And while a few studies have linked higher protein diets with increased satiety and weight loss, there is evidence that they are associated with decreased lifespan.[16]

Just like not all carbs are created equal, neither are all proteins. A diet composed of a mix of quality plant and animal protein from whole food sources differs from a diet of hotdogs, bacon, lunch meat, protein bars, and protein powders.

The manufacturer may claim a protein powder is vegan or that the bacon is from turkey, but that does not make it healthy. When in doubt, always remember Mother Nature trumps Nabisco and General Mills.

But I thought high-protein diets were good for weight loss?

All diets can be good for weight loss if you employ sufficient calorie restriction, at least in the short term. The problem is the foods we eat not only provide calories via macronutrients, but they also provide us with a smorgasbord of vitamins, minerals, phytonutrients, and fiber. Hopefully, by now, you are starting to appreciate why eating to lose weight is different from eating to support a lean, strong, and healthy body. A lean, strong, and healthy body is best supported by eating a variety of intact, quality foods, many of them plant-based.

There is evidence that adding a little extra protein to your meal may help with feelings of fullness and satiety. But that does not mean we need to consume the copious amounts suggested by pseudo-experts or that they should come from processed sources like protein powder.

Okay, but what if I'm diabetic?

As I mentioned before, diabetics also need to eat a diverse whole-foods-based diet that ideally includes all the macronutrients and the unique blend of micronutrients they provide. If you are sensitive to carbs, you may find that eating a little more protein can be beneficial. But this does not equate to simply upping your intake of processed meats and other pseudo-food protein sources, which is exactly what people do. It means eating quality sources of whole plant-based and animal proteins.

What about BCAAs?

BCAA is an acronym for branched-chain amino acids. They

include leucine, isoleucine, and valine, three of the nine essential amino acids.

I include a brief discussion of them here because they have recently become quite popular.

There is research that suggests taking BCAA supplements before exercise may decrease general fatigue and the breakdown of muscle. For this reason, BCAA supplementation has become more common. Unfortunately, not all studies agree. In several studies, supplementation with BCAA, at least in mice, decreased lifespan and increased obesity. It also increased glucose intolerance.[17] There is also some evidence of other negative health consequences, like a link to ALS.[18]

The problem with supplementing is that it may create an imbalance that has both positive and negative consequences. We just do not know. Yet this does not stop people desperate to achieve a lean physique from trying them. If the robust multi-billion-dollar supplement industry proves anything, it is that we love to put our faith in pills, powders, and potions.

Take Home Point:

Consuming a diet rich in quality complementary plant proteins and, to a lesser extent, animal protein will not only provide the amino acids we need but also all the other nutrients necessary to support health and fight disease.

Most people eating a whole foods diet will get all the protein they need without trying. This is because even plant foods like nuts, seeds, whole intact grains, legumes, beans, and lentils contain a decent amount of protein per serving. Add in fish, meat, eggs, and dairy, and most people are more than covered.

And just like the best sources of carbohydrates are intact minimally processed foods, so are the best sources of protein.

Finally, do not let the manufacturers of popular protein products like protein powders and processed meats dupe you, as they are likely no better than refined carbohydrates.

Fat

Dietary fats are the third group of macronutrients. Unlike carbs and protein, which both provide four calories of energy per gram, each gram of fat provides us with nine calories, which makes it a dense source of energy. Dietary fat is important thanks to its role in the absorption of the fat-soluble vitamins A, D, K and E. It is also necessary for supporting brain health and function and the production of healthy cholesterol. Though we often view cholesterol as bad, it has important roles in the body, which include maintaining cellular health and the production of important hormones.

Structurally speaking, fats contain a glycerol backbone and three fatty acid chains.

The fatty acid chains are further classified as monounsaturated, polyunsaturated, and saturated based on the number of double-bonded carbons. Individual fats are classified based on the predominant fatty acid composition.

Monounsaturated fats contain fatty acid chains with just one double-bonded carbon. Sources include nuts, avocados, olive oil, peanut oil, and canola oil.

Polyunsaturated fats contain fatty acid chains with more than one double bond. Examples include liquid cooking oils such as sunflower and safflower, nuts, seeds, and fatty fish.

Saturated fats contain no double bonds, and thus the carbons are saturated with hydrogens. Sources of saturated fat include animal and animal products, as well as coconut and palm oil.

Both mono- and polyunsaturated fats are of plant origin except for fish oils. Saturated fats are of animal origin, with a few exceptions like coconut oil (80 - 90 percent saturated fat) and palm oil (about 35 percent saturated).

The differences in a fat's chemical structure—the presence or absence of double bonded carbons—affect a fat's physical properties, such as whether it is a solid or liquid at room temperature and its smoke point (aka its burning point).

The more saturated a fat, the more solid it will be at room temperature and the higher the smoke point, making it a better choice for cooking at higher temperatures.

Their differences may also determine a fat's impact on our health.

Traditionally, experts believed that saturated fats were less healthy than unsaturated fats because they contributed to heart disease via their impact on LDL cholesterol. It was also believed that high-fat diets contributed to an increased risk of certain cancers. Heart disease and cancer continue to be major killers in the US and other developed countries. For this reason, experts recommended we limit the consumption of fat to 30 percent of our total caloric intake and saturated fat to under 10 percent.

These recommendations have been questioned and criticized over the past two decades. Several meta analyses suggest that fat, generally, and saturated fat, specifically, do not cause or contribute to heart disease and cancer.

The problem is the original recommendations were based primarily on epidemiological data. This type of data examines the frequency of disease in a particular culture with certain dietary patterns. Unfortunately, epidemiological data can establish a correlation but not necessarily a causation. And it turns out that while such studies can be useful for trying to understand the impact of a comprehensive lifestyle on certain disease processes; they are not always so helpful when evaluating the overall impact of individual nutrients like fat.

For example, it turns out not all saturated fats are created equal. So, the saturated fat in coconut butter may differ from the saturated fat found in a big juicy steak and for various reasons. What we replace the fat with (saturated or otherwise) may also matter. Historically, under the impression that fat was bad, people started eating more unhealthy processed carbs, which contribute to the development of lifestyle diseases, including heart disease and cancer. In short, we exchanged one evil for another.

The impact of fat and saturated fat on our health likely depends on the overall quality and composition of the diet, health status, activity level, and other lifestyle factors.

This said, when it comes to saturated fat, the jury is still out with most public health experts admitting that saturated fats are a grey area but then still sticking with the earlier conservative recommendation for limiting saturated fats to less than 10 percent of total calories (specifically when consumed as processed meats like lunch meat and bacon) while broadening their recommendations for fats generally.

That said, stay tuned!

Trans/Hydrogenated fats are another type of fat and an unhealthy product of the food industry in which food companies hydrogenated (infused with hydrogen) a polyunsaturated fat to produce a substance that is solid at room temperature. The idea was to create a healthier solid fat (margarine as a healthy alternative to butter). Only it turns out that these synthetic molecules are much worse than the saturated fats they were created to replace.

Another common classification of fats is the omega-3, omega-6, and omega-9 fatty acids, whose names are based on the position of the last double bond relative to the omega end. All are important for good health.

Omega-3 fatty acids are polyunsaturated fats whose last double bond occurs three carbons from the omega end of the molecule. They are essential because our body needs them but cannot make them, meaning we must get them from the diet.

Omega-3 fats are further classified as EPA, DHA, and ALA.

EPA or **eicosapentaenoic acid** is important in controlling inflammation.

DHA or **docosahexaenoic acid** is important for brain development and function.

ALA or **alpha-linoleic acid** is good for many organ systems. It can also be used to make EPA and DHA, though conversion rates are low and can vary depending on the overall quality of the diet.

EPA and DHA are present in fatty fish and are thus often referred to as fish oils.

ALA has a plant origin and can be found in flax, hemp, chia, walnuts, avocados, and the oils made from these foods.

There is currently a greater body of research that has established the benefits of fish oils. However, most experts believe that ALA offers similar benefits based on the studies conducted thus far.

Omega-6 fatty acids are polyunsaturated fats that contain their last double bond at the sixth carbon from the omega end of the molecule.

Like omega-3 fats, omega-6 fats are also essential and therefore must be garnered from the diet.

Omega-6 fats are used for energy and are also important in supporting immune system function via their role in making pro-inflammatory eicosanoids. In small amounts, these eicosanoids are important in the healing and immune responses, but in large quantities and not properly balanced with the effects of omega-3 fats, they may contribute to systemic inflammation.

In countries that consume too many processed foods, omega-6 fatty acids are in abundant supply, readily consumed, and too often out of proportion to omega-3 fats.

The ideal ratio of omega-6 fats to omega-3 fats is 4:1. In countries like the United States, we are consuming closer to 15:1 or more. This is because the refined oils used in processed foods are high in omega-6 fats. This combined with a low consumption of fish and plant foods high in ALA explains the imbalance.

Though many fitness/health professionals sing the praises of omega-3 fats, calling them anti-inflammatory, while cursing omega-6 fats, calling them pro-inflammatory, this is an oversimplification. Both omega-3 and omega-6 fats are essential and important for good health. Unfortunately, we are currently not balancing these two important nutrients in our diet. It is the imbalance rather than the nutrients themselves that is to blame.

Omega-9 fatty acids are monounsaturated fats in which the single double bond occurs nine carbons from the omega end of the fatty acid chain.

Unlike omega-3s and omega-6s, the body can synthesize omega-9 fatty acids, meaning they are important but not essential in the sense that we can make them if we need them.

Experts believe eating more omega-9 fatty acids, especially if they replace less healthy saturated fats, is a good thing.

What about taking omega 3/fish oil supplements?

I am not a fan of supplements, mainly because we really do not understand the long-term implications of taking them. Since I will cover my concerns regarding supplements in more detail later, I will just say now that my concerns about fish oil supplements do not differ from my concerns about supplements generally.

Take Home Point:

Dietary fat is an energy-dense macronutrient that is essential for good health. Though fats were once demonized, they have since been vindicated. Like all macronutrients, when it comes to fats, quality matters. Thus, the best source of fat is intact whole foods. And because there are still grey areas around saturated fat, the jury is still out about the role they should ultimately play in the diet with most conventional experts recommending we limit them to less than 10 percent of our total calorie intake.

Macronutrient Summary

Whether talking about carbohydrates, proteins, or fats the key is the quality more so than the quantity. Whole intact food sources are not only superior nutritionally speaking, but they also do not appear to have the same detrimental effects on our health as heavily processed foods. Whole foods, in general, refer to those foods you could raise or grow on the farm. They have been minimally processed and are close to their natural form.

Regarding ideal macronutrient ratios in the diet, if one exists, that ratio is not well-established or universally accepted. It may be helpful to manipulate the amount of each macronutrient that goes beyond just choosing quality sources, although much of what pseudo experts recommend lacks any scientific support or evidence.

What does seem to be worthwhile is eating a variety of quality carbohydrates, protein, and fat sources, mainly from plant foods every day and even every meal. This will ensure that not only do you get a good mix of the macronutrients you need but also a good mix of vitamins, minerals, phytonutrients, and fiber.

The best overall macronutrient breakdown, if one does exist, may depend on your age, activity level, underlying health conditions, sex, preference, fitness/performance goals, and palatability among other potential factors.

UNDERSTANDING GUT HEALTH

"We inherit every one of our genes, but we leave the womb without a single microbe. As we pass through our mother's birth canal, we attract entire colonies of bacteria. By the time a child can crawl, he has been blanketed by an enormous unseen cloud of microorganisms--a hundred trillion or more. They are bacteria, mostly, but also viruses and fungi (including a variety of yeast), and they come at us from all directions: other people, food, furniture, clothing, cars, buildings, trees, pets, even the air we breathe. They congregate in our digestive systems and our mouths, fill the space between our teeth, cover our skin, and line our throats. We are inhabited by as many as ten thousand bacterial species; those cells outnumber those which we consider our own by ten to one and weigh about three pounds—the same as our brain. Together they are referred to as our microbiome--and they play such a crucial role in our lives that scientists like [Martin J.] Blaser have begun to reconsider what it means to be human."

MICHAEL SPECTER

T hanks to the microscope, theories about small unseen organisms were first confirmed in the second half of the 17th century.

Robert Hooke would describe the fruiting structure of molds in 1665, followed by Antoni van Leeuwenhoek, who is credited with the discovery of bacteria in 1676.

But it was the German bacteriologist Robert Koch, also known as the father of microbiology, who—almost two-hundred years later—showed that microscopic bacteria were the cause behind infectious diseases like anthrax, tuberculosis, and cholera.

Then in the 1920s, British scientist Alexander Fleming discovered the first antibiotic while working in his laboratory in London. One of the greatest discoveries of the 20th century, the impetus for our first antibiotic occurred when Fleming observed that mold growing on the same plate slowed the growth of Staphylococcus aureus bacteria.

This observation would spur two decades of research that ultimately resulted in penicillin, the first-ever antibiotic.

Unfortunately, when we think of bacteria, funguses, or viruses, we often think exclusively of sickness, disease, and even death rather than health, wellness, and longevity. Yet not only can microorganisms be detrimental to our health in certain situations, they can also be essential to it.

Thanks to the field of microbiology and the human microbiome project, we are finally beginning to fully appreciate the significant contributions that the human microbiome makes to our health. Interestingly, the microbes that live on and in us outnumber human cells and contribute significantly more DNA toward our health than our own human genes.

For instance, microbes in the colon can digest fiber we cannot, producing short-chain fatty acids which are believed to not only be important in gut health but also exert a critical influence over many organs, including the brain.

Likewise, researchers have linked a less diverse microbiome in mice with obesity and a more diverse microbiome with leanness. Interestingly, obese mice could be made leaner simply by introducing them to a more diverse microbiome, but only if they ate a healthy chow (described as low in saturated fat and high in fruits and veggies).[19]

Additionally, a better understanding of the microbiome may also help explain the negative health consequences attributed to red meat that goes beyond saturated fat. Some researchers have postulated that a carbohydrate called N-glycolylneuraminic acid (Neu5Gc), a sugar found in meat that our bodies can no longer produce but that can be incorporated into our cells if eaten in the diet, is partly to blame. Researchers believe our immune system recognizes Neu5Gc as foreign and produces antibodies against it, contributing to systemic inflammation and inflammatory diseases. Recent research conducted at the University of California, San Diego found genetically altered mice that could also not produce Neu5Gc and that were fed diets high in red meat had a decrease in microbiome diversity and an increase in enzymes associated with the release of Neu5Gc.[20]

In other words, a diet high in red meat may alter the microbiome in such a way as to encourage the release of Neu5Gc, a sugar that when incorporated into our cells may contribute to inflammation and inflammatory lifestyle diseases.

While our understanding of the microbiome and its influence on us increases daily, it is still in its infancy. If you are interested in learning more, I would recommend reading *The Human Superorganism* by Rodney Dietert, PhD as a starting point. Unfortunately, while it is a fascinating topic, it goes well beyond the focus and scope of this book.

For our discussion here in this limited space, I would like to talk about diet, exercise, and other lifestyle choices as they relate to the microbiome.

Interestingly, a cursory review of the current science suggests that what is good for us is also good for our microbiome, which makes complete sense since it would seem a healthy body is and always has depended on a healthy microbiome and vice versa.

For example, a plant-based, whole foods diet that is high in fiber supports our general health because it also supports a healthy microbiome, which I hope you are beginning to appreciate is an essential part of us. Regular exercise and adequate sleep, too, seem to play important roles in promoting a mix of healthy microbes in our personal ecosystem and supporting our health.

What about taking probiotics and prebiotics?

A **probiotic** is a food or supplement that contains a live active bacterial culture. Foods that contain probiotics include fermented foods like yogurt, sauerkraut, kefir, kimchi, kombucha, pickles, tempeh, and miso. In addition, there are currently a number of supplements or nonfood sources of probiotics available.

A **prebiotic** is food for those microbes, such as the undigestible fiber found in plant foods.

Because microbiome diversity is considered good for us, the idea behind consuming foods or supplements with probiotics and/or prebiotics is to increase that diversity. It is also championed as a way to repopulate an altered microbiome that results from a sickness or a course of antibiotics.

Only like most things, what seems simple on the surface rarely is. The problem is we just do not know how much is enough or what constitutes healthy or if there are multiple possibilities. And even if we did, simply taking a supplement or food with a particular probiotic—as in the experiment with obese mice referenced above—may not matter unless we also address the overall quality of diet and/or other lifestyle factors that support that microbiome.

Simply eating a healthy plant-based diet, exercising regularly, and getting adequate rest may be the best way to promote and maintain your specific healthy microbiome and a healthy body.

Take Home Point:

We are not simply a body. We are an ecosystem, a diverse collection of human cells, bacterial cells, funguses, and even viruses, all living together in/on this thing we call our body. What we eat, how we move, and even how we sleep combined with our human genome, can affect our microbiome just as our microbiome can affect us.

What is good for us is coincidentally good for the bugs that live in and on us.

Beyond that, it is just not clear, which means taking a probiotic or a prebiotic is not necessarily helpful, or if it is, it may be purely by chance. So rather than running out and buying the newest probiotic supplement, it might be better to focus on those behaviors that not only support our health but likely do so because they support a healthy microbiome, which may look a little different for everyone. Any claim to the contrary is simply good marketing.

Eating a plant-heavy, fiber-rich diet that emphasizes whole foods, moving regularly in ways that support overall health, sleeping well, and managing stress are not only strategies for promoting overall good health but also for cultivating a healthy microbiome.

SUPPLEMENTS
- TO TAKE OR
NOT TO TAKE

"Nutritional supplements are not a substitute for a nutritionally balanced diet."

DEEPAK CHOPRA

O ur obsession with supplements, buying them, taking them, and promoting them is nothing short of mindboggling.

Maybe it is our desire to find the magic pill that will not only keep us healthy but also looking and feeling younger, or maybe we are a distributor for an MLM trying to make a little side cash. Whatever the case, our love affair with supplements is evident in the multi-billion-dollar industry they have become.

Having been part of the fitness industry for over thirty years, I have seen hundreds of supplements come and go. Early on, I even took a few.

I understand the temptation to pop a pill that promises health or leanness. I get it. Unfortunately, supplements and the way most people use them is concerning, and so I have devoted an entire chapter in this book to discussing them.

By definition, a dietary supplement is a product that increases the amount of a particular nutrient and/or substance in a diet. They can have a couple ingredients extracted from natural foods and packaged in another form or they can contain multiple ingredients, which may be synthetic. Examples include vitamin and mineral supplements, protein powders, amino acids, herbal supplements, fish oils, collagen supplements, probiotics, prebiotics, and a never-ending slew of supposed performance enhancers.

In the US, the FDA regulates dietary supplements as food, so they are subject to general quality, packaging, and labeling criteria. Yet, unlike pharmaceuticals, they are not reviewed and approved based on safety and effectiveness. What this means is that they undergo a much less rigorous vetting than traditional pharmaceuticals, even though they often claim to provide a medicinal effect and even though ingredients may interact with prescription drugs.

This does not mean a supplement is dangerous, but just that it is not held to the same standard as traditional pharmaceuticals, which may or may not be a problem for the person taking it.

More concerning is that too many people take supplements blindly based on a blurb they read on the internet, something they heard about at the gym, or a recommendation from a friend. For example, they may know someone who takes iron and who claims it gives them more energy. So, without a clue about their own iron status, they take a supplement, too.

They may or may not have a low iron status and taking the supplement may or may not have beneficial effects. And even if taking a supplement appears to help, the observed effect may or may not result from the supplement but instead from the placebo effect. Often when we believe something will work, it does, and vice versa. But more notably, the actual effect may be detrimental, if not in the short term, then in the long term.

The problem is we rarely know the negative effects of dietary supplements, especially with prolonged or long-term usage.

Not only do many supplements not have the desired effects we believe them to, but they may also cause unwanted side effects.

For example, blindly taking supplements has the potential to create an imbalance. We already know that having too much of one nutrient may impact the absorption and utilization of another.

When we talked about omega fats, I pointed out that both omega-3 fats and omega-6 fats are essential, but when imbalanced in the diet the way they are in the American diet, omega-6 fats can be proinflammatory.

An imbalance in nutrients is often just as concerning as a deficiency.

Unfortunately, supplements, unlike pharmaceuticals, often get a free pass. The assumption is that even if they do not deliver on their promises, there are no downsides to taking them. Only research tells us this is not necessarily the case.

A notable example involves mega doses of the antioxidants vitamin A, vitamin E, and vitamin C. Back in the '80s, we not only believed large doses of these antioxidants to be safe because of their low toxicity, but we also believed they were protective against cancer and stroke. Yet, over the years scientists have linked lung cancer, prostate cancer, and at least one type of stroke to large doses of antioxidants.

This illustrates how taking supplements blindly and assuming they are safe is naive.

Even when prescribed, supplements may still not be safe. For example, once touted as an effective treatment for high cholesterol, large doses of the B vitamin niacin were prescribed by doctors as a therapy to raise HDL (good cholesterol). Yet, while niacin raised HDL, it did not seem to impact the rate of death from a heart attack or stroke. Additionally, there were serious potential side effects linked to the prescription supplements, such as elevated blood sugars, strokes, bleeding, liver damage, and even infection. And while these large doses are sold only via prescription, it still highlights why taking nutrients out of the context of food may not be as helpful or as safe as we assume.

Another example is calcium supplements. Experts once believed that taking calcium, with or without vitamin D, could decrease the risk of fracture as we age. Only a more recent meta-analysis suggests that not only is there a marginal benefit to calcium supplementation regarding fracture risk, but also that taking calcium supplements increases the risk of cardiovascular events in healthy older women, a demographic for which the supplement is routinely recommended.[21] This is not true of dietary calcium consumed through food, suggesting that the bolus calcium entering the bloodstream via supplement form may be the issue, although there is still a lot we don't know. Now I am not suggesting someone who is taking calcium under a doctor's guidance should stop taking it, but I am suggesting that all of us, including health professionals, should be more thoughtful when weighing the risks and benefits of a supplement, particularly one that is taken for a long period.

The bottom line is that people often take supplements whose long-term effects are poorly understood even if they deliver in the short term—a big *if* since many supplements make claims that lack evidence. They also have no basis to objectively and critically evaluate/measure a supplement's impact on their various body systems.

Furthermore, most nutrients taken in supplemental form occur in real food. Time and time again, getting nutrients through food is not only safer but also more effective.

For example, taking a vitamin C supplement to ward off the flu is arguably inferior to eating an orange, which not only provides a natural source of vitamin C, but also fiber that feeds our microbiome (now understood to be critical to our immune system function). Eating the orange also provides other important nutrients and micronutrients important for general health. Finally, the orange may displace a less healthy, pro-inflammatory food in the diet.

The belief that supplements are safe is inherently flawed, as there are many notable examples in the scientific literature that contradict this assumption.

It should come as no surprise then that the bulk of people promoting supplements usually have little education in the nutritional sciences or even the health sciences. Worse, they are sometimes selling the very thing they are promoting. Even most doctors and other trained and licensed health professionals have little to no training in nutrition.

Remember, supplements are a multi-billion-dollar industry, yet we are fatter and sicker than ever.

Additionally, those selling supplements often use untrue claims to convince us we need what they are selling. For example, I was once told by a colleague selling a popular nutritional product that the fruits and veggies we eat are nutritionally inferior to the same fruits and veggies of yesteryear and thus incapable of providing the nutrition we need. This is a common claim made by various supplement companies as it is an effective marketing/sales strategy. And while it is probably true that current farming and distribution practices result in a product that is marginally inferior to the locally grown produce of years ago, the data would suggest that we are not getting fat and sick because our produce is nutritionally inferior to the produce of our grandparents. We are getting fat and sick because less than 10 percent of us are eating even the minimum daily recommended servings of fruits and veggies.

On another occasion, I was told by the rep of a popular MLM (multi-level marketing) company trying to recruit me and another nutritional professional that we should not worry if we knew nothing about nutrition (although, unlike him, we both had degrees in nutrition) because neither did he when he first started selling the product. After the meeting, I took the huge and professional-looking info packet and researched the studies they cited to support their product, only to find that not one said what the company claimed it did.

Not even close.

Should I ever take a supplement?

Like most answers I will give in this book, *it depends*. Just like there is a time and place for traditional pharmaceuticals, there may be a time and place for supplements.

For example, a particular supplement may offer the same benefits as a pharmaceutical, but at a slightly lower risk and/or lower cost, although the true risk of supplements is often unknown or not well established.

Another case might be where an underlying deficiency exists that would be hard to treat via diet alone.

And finally, one might opt for a supplement where the risks (both known and unknown) are worth it to the individual. An example might be BCAAs. The consumption of branched-chain amino acids prior to exercise or an athletic event might delay fatigue and decrease muscle breakdown, and for an athlete, this could mean the difference between winning and losing and thus worth the potential risk.

If you do take supplements, do so judiciously and with a healthy amount of skepticism and the realization that they may not always be safe or do what they claim to do.

And keep in mind that supplements often give us a false sense of security, which allows us to ignore or skimp on other proven behaviors that are essential to good health.

Despite marketing claims to the contrary, supplements will never be a replacement for healthy eating habits or other healthy behaviors like getting adequate exercise and sleep.

Take Home Point:

Supplements are big money, probably because they appeal to our desire for a magic pill. But not only do they not always do what they claim, they may cause harm when taken blindly.

Assuming a supplement works is naive, but assuming it is safe could be dangerous. If you must take a supplement, do your research, and do not simply stop on the first page of Google.

Also, make sure you have some objective way to measure if the supplement is having the desired effect.

Finally, remember that supplements will never replace a balanced diet or other healthy behaviors like regular movement and quality sleep no matter how seductive and sexy the marketing claims.

HORMONES

E ver been told you need to balance your hormones? Do you even have an inkling of what that means, or how to go about balancing them in the first place?

While there is a lot of talk about hormones as they relate to weight, weight loss, weight gain, and even health, very few people understand what supporting hormonal health looks like, although it makes for a savvy and seductive marketing campaign from a fitness industry that is always searching for ways to repackage its newest weight-loss message.

Yet, sale's strategies aside, hormones are indeed important. Chemical messengers within the body, they regulate the various body systems, including metabolism, homeostasis, sexual function, growth and development, mood, reproduction, and the sleep-wake cycle.

Understanding hormones and what can impact them can go a long way toward helping us better appreciate the nuances and impact of our lifestyle choices on both our weight and our health.

Several organs produce over fifty known hormones, including the pituitary gland, the hypothalamus, the pineal gland, the thyroid and the parathyroid, the pancreas, the ovaries and testes, the adrenal glands, the liver, the kidneys, and the gut. Even adipose tissue, though once believed to be inert tissue, produces hormones such as leptin, estrogen, and adiponectin.

Hormones play a critical role in health as too little or too much of a hormone or the inability of the body to respond to a hormone can cause serious problems. They may also play a significant role in weight gain and difficulty losing weight.

For example, hormones like insulin, leptin, ghrelin, cortisol, and estrogen may not only be making us fat but keeping us that way.

Insulin

Produced by the pancreas in response to a post-meal rise in blood sugar, **insulin** is an anabolic hormone that transports glucose and the energy from our food into the liver, fat, and muscle cells, where it is either metabolized for energy or stored as fat or glycogen for later use.

Insulin is often described as a key that unlocks the cell, allowing glucose in.

When insulin levels are high, the liver stops making and releasing glucose into the blood. Vice versa, when insulin levels are low because blood glucose levels are low, it triggers the release of glucagon, a hormone that regulates catabolic processes and favors the release of stored energy by signaling the liver to pump glucose into the bloodstream via the mobilization of glycogen or fat reserves.

Large and frequent insulin spikes contribute to insulin resistance, a condition in which the body is producing insulin but is less effective because the cells have become resistant or less sensitive to it. Using the key analogy above, the key no longer fits the lock it is supposed to open, in which case the cell remains closed and blood sugars remain high. Over time, insulin resistance can lead to diseases like metabolic syndrome and type 2 diabetes, both characterized by chronic hyperglycemia (elevated blood sugar).

These chronically elevated blood glucose levels, best measured by an AC1, can damage organs like the kidneys, blood vessels, the eyes, and even the nerves. They also contribute to chronic systemic inflammation, a risk factor for chronic lifestyle diseases, including heart disease, cancer, and

Alzheimer's.

Obesity and overweight are both considered risk factors for insulin resistance. Likewise, many experts believe that chronically elevated insulin levels secondary to specific dietary patterns (eating poor quality calories, eating too many calories, and eating too often throughout the day) may contribute to insulin resistance, weight gain, obesity, and difficulty losing weight. Other non-diet-related factors like inadequate sleep, lack of exercise, and stress can also affect insulin sensitivity both in the short and long term. Finally, because the female hormones estrogen and progesterone affect insulin function, the changes in these hormones associated with perimenopause and menopause may contribute to a decline in insulin sensitivity as we age.

Insulin resistance exists along a spectrum, so even those who do not meet the criteria for pre-diabetes or diabetes may still overproduce insulin in an effort to regulate blood glucose levels. When the keys do not work or do not work well, our body may keep making more keys to open the locks. Unfortunately, elevated levels of insulin resulting in insulin resistance leads to even higher levels of insulin. It is a vicious circle.

Understanding the role of insulin and its impact on weight and health can be an important part of both achieving and maintaining a healthy body. As we mentioned previously, if insulin levels are high, it inhibits the release of glucagon. In turn, this may affect fat storage and fat utilization, ultimately affecting weight gain or difficulty with losing weight.

Luckily, we can support optimal insulin function by eating high-quality whole foods (intact whole grains, fruits, veggies, beans, lentils, legumes, nuts, seeds, and quality lean meat), exercising regularly, sleeping well, and managing stress effectively. There is also evidence that fasting, whether just increasing the overnight fast or engaging in a longer sustained fasting period that may span several days, is an effective and viable strategy for improving insulin sensitivity and preventing or even reversing insulin resistance. In cases, where someone is already insulin resistent, a lower carb diet may offer some additional benefits, at least in the short term.

Leptin

Though we once believed adipose to be inert tissue, we now understand that fat stored in the body secretes important hormones. Leptin is one such hormone.

Only recently discovered in 1994 by Douglas Coleman and Jeffrey Friedman, leptin plays a key role in regulating body weight and our energy balance. Leptin inhibits pathways that stimulate food intake. It also increases metabolism. In this way, leptin helps to regulate energy consumption and energy storage.

Sometimes referred to as the satiety hormone, leptin increases in the fed state and decreases in the fasting state, while overall leptin levels also reflect fat stores so that more stored fat results in higher leptin output. In short, when leptin levels are high, it signals to our brain that we have eaten enough. It also tells the body it is okay to burn stored energy. Vice versa, when leptin levels are low, it signals the body to eat more and to hold on to stored energy by lowering energy output.

Worth noting is that the impact of too much leptin appears muted when compared to too little. Our bodies evolved to protect us preferentially and vigorously from getting too thin as opposed to getting too fat. This makes sense when you consider that having inadequate fat stores was historically a threat whereas having too much fat was not. Unfortunately, thanks to our modern lifestyles, this has changed, but our physiology has not.

After discovering leptin and identifying its role in energy balance, scientists wondered if a leptin deficiency or a malfunction of the leptin receptors might explain obesity, further postulating that treatment with leptin might cure obesity. This possibility was considered after scientists identified that a genetic disorder resulting in a leptin deficiency caused extreme hunger, overeating, and severe obesity in children who, once treated with leptin, were finally able to reach and maintain a healthy weight.

Unfortunately, though a handful of obese individuals do possess a genetic or acquired condition that affects leptin production and/or function, leptin alone is not the only factor impacting most overweight and obese individuals. Much to Big Pharma's dismay, leptin therapy as a cure for obesity was a total bust.

Another potential issue with the leptin feedback loop is something called *leptin resistance.* Just like repeated exposure to elevated insulin levels can decrease a cell's insulin sensitivity, prolonged exposure to high leptin levels results in a decreased leptin sensitivity. It is possible that over time the body adopts a new normal with respect to leptin, thus impairing the leptin feedback loop in a way that favors more fat storage or a higher set point/range.

Interestingly, chronically high insulin levels not only cause insulin resistance but also appear to cause leptin resistance.

The question then becomes *how does one increase leptin sensitivity or reset the baseline?* Sadly, the answer is unknown. Not gaining weight in the first place would be ideal, but not necessarily practical for someone who is already overweight.

Still, there may be things you can do to improve leptin sensitivity. For example, a handful of studies have found that getting adequate sleep (eight to ten hours) decreases leptin resistance, as does regular exercise.

Our dietary patterns may also play a role. Several animal models suggest that certain macronutrient profiles may help either decrease or increase leptin resistance. For example, higher-fat diets—especially those high in omega-6 fats and high in carbohydrates like fructose—were linked to increased leptin resistance, while diets with at least 20 percent of calories coming from protein seemed to decrease resistance.

While it is tempting to extrapolate studies in mice to humans, it may be naïve to do so, and this is an area where more research is needed before drawing conclusions.

Finally, calorie restriction, at least in the short term, appeared to improve leptin resistance, though longer-term studies suggest that weight loss is the actual key. Of course, these findings, too, are preliminary, and there is a lot we still do not understand.[22]

The real take-home point is that the energy balance equation (calories in versus calories out) is a little more complicated than most people realize. Hormones, like leptin, play a role that goes beyond a calorie surplus or calorie deficit. Our metabolic health is a factor in weight gain, weight loss and maintaining a healthy weight that may be independent of calories, and there are many things—both internal and external—that may affect our metabolic health.

Several lifestyle factors likely come into play only we do not understand all the nuances. In the end, there may be a reason some people struggle more than others with achieving and maintaining a healthy level of leanness that extends beyond the oversimplified calories in versus calories out model. Eating too many calories is a problem, but hormones like leptin strongly influence how much we eat. And a multitude of factors may affect leptin levels and leptin sensitivity.

Ghrelin

If leptin is the satiety hormone, then ghrelin is the hunger hormone. Scientists believe ghrelin plays a role in stimulating hunger as blood levels rise shortly before a meal. Though not completely understood, an empty stomach triggers the release of this hormone from cells, primarily in the stomach.

As expected, calorie-restricted diets lead to increases in ghrelin. What is less expected is that ghrelin levels appear to stay elevated long after the diet ends. In fact, increases in post dieting ghrelin may help to explain why so many people regain the weight. With higher levels of circulating ghrelin, you stay hungry and are more likely to overeat.

On the other hand, ghrelin is often lower in obese individuals, leading to speculation that this population has an increased sensitivity to the hormone. At least one study found that ghrelin levels also did not fall significantly after a meal in obese subjects when compared to lean subjects, suggesting that ghrelin levels are already maximally suppressed in this group. Since ghrelin increases to stimulate hunger and decreases after a meal for several hours to decrease or inhibit hunger, ghrelin remaining low would suggest that this feedback loop is not working or working optimally in obese individuals. Finally, those who have undergone gastric bypass have lower ghrelin levels. These lower levels may account for the higher success rates in this population regarding keeping off the weight once lost.[23]

Again, there is still much we do not know about the impact of hormones like leptin and ghrelin on weight gain, weight loss, and weight maintenance. But, once again, what does seem clear is that our bodies are not closed systems in which calories in and calories out are universally fixed or even easily calculated by some fitness app. Hormones can have a substantial impact on the *calories in* via their control of hunger and satiety and on *calories out* via their ability to both ramp up and slow down our metabolism.

It also appears that behaviors that support our general health, adequate sleep, healthy eating patterns, stress management, and achieving and maintaining a healthy weight all support optimal ghrelin and leptin levels and function.

Cortisol

Often referred to as the stress hormone, cortisol is a glucocorticoid—or steroid hormone—released in response to stress, including acute, chronic, and traumatic stress.

Almost every organ system in the body has glucocorticoid receptors, meaning high or low cortisol levels can impact their function.

Under stressful situations, our adrenal glands release cortisol as part of the fight-or-flight response. Unlike insulin which clears glucose from the bloodstream, cortisol signals the liver to pump more sugar into the system to prepare for dealing with a perceived threat. In this way, cortisol can contribute to chronically elevated blood glucose levels. Cortisol also decreases insulin sensitivity.

In small doses, such as those that result from temporary stresses like exercise or even fasting, cortisol decreases overall inflammation. However, in larger doses, such as those seen with chronic physical or emotional stress, cortisol can lead to chronic systemic inflammation, compromising immune system function, and contributing to lifestyle diseases like high blood pressure and heart disease.

Cortisol naturally spikes in the morning and decreases throughout the day and is known to help regulate the sleep-wake cycle. Elevated cortisol levels negatively affect sleep. Likewise, poor sleep can lead to elevated cortisol levels. Another vicious cycle.

Cortisol also favors weight gain in the abdomen. Since levels of the stress hormone increase starting in our forties (often peaking during menopause) elevated cortisol may help to explain changes in the sleep-wake cycle seen as we age as well as the tendency to put on weight around the middle in midlife.

Finally, the elevated cortisol levels associated with prolonged stress not only increase appetite but also contribute to cravings for high-fat and high-sugar foods. Thus, too much cortisol may play a significant role in overeating, overweight, and obesity in some people.[24],[25]

Getting adequate sleep and regular exercise, limiting stress, breathing deeply, and even laughing can all help to prevent the unhealthy cortisol levels associated with chronic stress.

Estrogen and Progesterone

As women age, many complain it is easier to gain weight and harder to lose weight. They blame their weight gain on perimenopause and menopause and the changing levels of the hormones estrogen and progesterone experienced during these life stages.

Evidence, however, suggests that while the hormonal fluctuations women undergo as they age can affect their bodies in significant ways, these hormones' role in overweight and obesity is often exaggerated, an idea we will explore in this section. In reality, the struggle with weight during perimenopause and menopause is likely the result of several different age-related and lifestyle factors, and not necessarily or exclusively changes in their sex hormones.

During adolescence the sex hormone estrogen influences the development of female sex characteristics associated with puberty, while progesterone is important in regulating a woman's cycle and preparing the uterus for pregnancy.

After the onset of puberty, the amount of estrogen and progesterone varies throughout the menstrual cycle, which encompasses the first day of a woman's period and ends with the first day of her next period (approximately twenty-four to thirty-eight days).

The *follicular phase* makes up the first phase of the ovarian cycle of the menstrual cycle and begins on the first day of a woman's period and ends after ovulation. Toward the end of a period, a dominant follicle in one ovary produces more estrogen, which peaks just before ovulation.

The *proliferative phase* of the uterine cycle overlaps the follicular phase, starting on the last day of a woman's period and lasting until ovulation. During this time, the uterine lining thickens in response to increased estrogen levels.

About midway through the menstrual cycle, estrogen levels reach a threshold that triggers an increase in luteinizing

151

hormone, leading to ovulation or the release of an egg.

The *luteal phase* makes up the second phase of the ovarian cycle. During this phase, the follicle that released the egg becomes the corpus luteum, a structure that will continue to produce estrogen but that also produces progesterone. If a fertilized egg implants in the uterine wall, progesterone will support the early pregnancy. If the egg remains unfertilized, the corpus luteum breaks down, causing both estrogen and progesterone levels to dip, ultimately leading to menstruation (the period).

The *secretory phase* of the uterine cycle overlaps the luteal phase. As progesterone rises during this phase, it signals for the uterine lining to stop thickening and instead prepare for a pregnancy. If the egg is not fertilized, then the decrease in both progesterone and estrogen along with other changes associated with this phase causes blood vessels to constrict and the uterine lining to shed, thus starting the entire menstrual cycle over again.

It is worth noting here that besides leptin, adipose also produces estrogen. Thus, being overweight or obese can lead to excessively high estrogen levels that can negatively affect a woman's cycle and her fertility. On the other hand, having inadequate fat stores, such as those often seen in elite female athletes, can lead to low estrogen levels. These low levels can disrupt a woman's natural cycle, leading to amenorrhea, or the absence of menses.

Besides its critical role in regulating the menstrual cycle, estrogen also affects the urinary tract, the heart, the blood vessels, the brain, and the bones. For example, estrogen plays a role in bone resorption and may also be responsible for why very lean women experience thinning of their bones regardless of age.

As women age, they produce less estrogen. The initial decline in estrogen leads to a transitional phase known as perimenopause. Though this stage can start in a woman's thirties, the average onset is early to mid-forties. During these years, women may notice symptoms such as irregular periods, mood swings, vaginal dryness, and hot flashes, all the result of declining estrogen levels.

Perimenopause can last just a few years or for several years and symptoms can range from mild to severe.

A woman reaches menopause when she has gone a full year without a period. Post-menopause starts immediately and is a term sometimes used interchangeably with menopause.

Many women blame weight gain in their forties, fifties, and sixties on perimenopause and menopause. However, the changing hormones may not be the primary cause of weight gain.

In fact, there is evidence to suggest that much of the weight gain experienced during middle age is a consequence of the aging process and a whole slew of behavioral and lifestyle changes associated with age.

For example, from thirty years on, we are losing up to 3 percent of our lean body mass a year. Less lean tissue means fewer calories needed to maintain our weight. In short, our metabolism slows down, especially if we are not exercising regularly. Furthermore, reduced activity later in life is not uncommon and can be due to aging joints, health problems, and the increasing life commitments that often lead to healthy behaviors becoming less of a priority. Women in their forties and fifties are often juggling busy schedules that include careers and families. Finding time to exercise and eat healthy can be tough.

Inadequate or poor quality sleep and excess stress can also be factors.

Finally, women become more insulin resistant as they age independent of hormonal changes.

So, while it is possible that a decrease in the female sex hormones estrogen and progesterone may contribute to weight gain in midlife, it is just one factor among many and likely not even the biggest factor. The healthy behaviors outlined previously, things like eating seven to eight servings of fruits and veggies a day, limiting added sugar, increasing the overnight fast, moving daily, and getting adequate sleep all support hormone health throughout the lifecycle, including during perimenopause and menopause.

Summary

Hormones have an impact on all body systems including the metabolic system. As a result, hormones can impact weight and weight gain. Furthermore, weight and weight gain can impact hormones. But other lifestyle factors such as nutrition, sleep, stress, and movement play an even bigger role. In the end, balancing your hormones is often nothing more than engaging in behaviors that support your overall health.

EATING STRATEGIES

I f you hear me say it once, you will hear me say it multiple times. Diets rarely work. More often than not, they are a short-term change in eating patterns (aka a temporary fix) as opposed to a sustainable long-term eating strategy. They do not teach people how to eat to support leanness over the long haul. They teach them how to count and restrict calories but they rarely provide the forever strategy needed to stay lean, strong, and healthy for more than a hiccup.

In contrast, an eating strategy implies a methodical approach to eating that supports long-term health and wellness goals not just for a few weeks or a few months, but for forever. And it is not necessarily focused exclusively on weight loss, but instead on building a lean, strong, and healthy body.

There are many ways to eat strategically. Some have fancy names like Keto, Intermittent Fasting, or the Mediterranean Diet. And others are a unique blend of the various eating philosophies. Some have no name at all and reflect a personal preference.

Decades of research suggests any number of different strategies can result in success if the strategy is sustainable and supports health over the long haul.

In the following section, I explore common eating strategies, what they entail, their pros and cons, and why they may or may not be a viable and effective strategy for you at a particular point in time. Exploring the benefits and drawbacks of various eating practices will hopefully allow you to choose a strategy or strategies that work best for you.

SHAUN TAYLOR BEVINS

Keto

Keto—short for the ketogenic diet—is a very low-carb/high-fat diet introduced in the early 1900s to mimic the benefits of fasting, which had been used to treat epileptic seizures in children since at least 500 B.C. And it worked. Children following the diet often saw a marked decrease in the number of seizures.[26]

Yet, with the discovery of anti-seizure medications, the ketogenic diet became increasingly obsolete. Little is written about the ketogenic diet in medical journals until its reemergence following an NBC-TV's Dateline production about a young two-year-old boy named Charlie. Based on his son's success with the diet, Charlie's father formed the Charlie Foundation that would fund additional research, ultimately helping to re-establish the ketogenic diet as a valid treatment option for controlling seizures in children with epilepsy.

So how did a diet developed to prevent seizures in epileptic children become a popular weight loss strategy?

Well, first we need to talk about **ketosis**. Significantly limiting carbohydrates (under ten to fifteen grams/day) depletes glycogen stores (one way your body stores energy) and leaves the body no choice but to burn stored fat for fuel. As you might guess, any eating strategy that promises to burn fat will be a darling of the diet industry.

A Keto diet involves eating 70-80 percent of your calories from fat, 20-25 percent from protein, and about 5-10 percent from carbs. This breakdown may vary slightly depending on the source. Ideally, the fat and protein sources should come from high-quality, minimally refined food sources.

Though severe carbohydrate restriction will force the body to burn fat for fuel, contemporary Keto supporters often overlook the fact that the fat you are burning is often dietary fat as opposed to stored fat. This is because you will not burn stored fat until you have created a calorie deficit. Remember, calories do matter, even if they are not the only thing that does.

That said, the satiating effects of a very high-fat diet combined with severe carb restriction that often results in eating significantly fewer processed foods generally leads to an improvement in blood sugar, insulin sensitivity, and hunger, at least in the short term if only because it improves the overall quality of food being consumed. In fact, it is very possible that the benefits associated with the Keto diet may have less to do with ketosis and more to do with restricting processed foods.

It is also worth noting that almost all diets promote weight loss, largely because when people implement a new eating strategy, they end up restricting the amount or type of calories regardless of the macronutrient content of the diet. And as we have already established, calorie restriction will promote short-term weight loss and improved health metrics even if success is short-lived.

Regardless of the reason people lose weight on Keto, when put head-to-head against low-fat diets, several recent meta-analyses have indeed found that for the time frames studied, Keto may be superior with respect to promoting weight loss. A Keto diet may also provide additional benefits to those who are obese and/or have type 2 diabetes (those who are metabolically sick) thanks to the detrimental effects of insulin resistance and its impact on processing carbs.

That is the good news.

The bad news is that researchers have not studied the Keto diet over prolonged periods to determine if there are long-term negative consequences to severely limiting carbohydrates. For example, any eating strategy which restricts one of the macronutrients can lead to micronutrient deficiencies over time, particularly if quality whole foods do not replace the banned macronutrient. And if history has taught us anything, what we eat is often more important than what we restrict. For example, the low-fat craze of the

1980s-90s centered around fears about fat making us fat. This led to a robust campaign to restrict fat in the diet. The problem was we replaced the fat with nutritionally inferior, sugar-laden, reduced-fat products and not with healthy, whole-food carbohydrate sources.

The same is true with Keto. If you simply replace your carb-heavy Hostess Ho-Hos with highly processed pseudo foods like hotdogs, you are not doing your health or your weight any favors over the long term.

Another problem with restrictive diets is that they are associated with poor long-term compliance. Committing to a carb-restrictive diet like Keto is not for the faint of heart. Of course, it is possible to use a strategy like Keto as a springboard of sorts, particularly if you are insulin resistant as long as you eventually learn how to eat in a way that not only supports your goals but that is also sustainable.

Pros

- May produce greater weight loss than a traditional low-fat diet, at least initially
- Seems to offer additional benefits to those who are obese, have diabetes, or are insulin resistant
- Can lead to decreased hunger thanks to the satiating effects of a high-fat diet
- Can improve the overall quality of diet, particularly if quality fats replace low-quality, refined carbs

Cons

- Though believed to be safe when healthy food choices are made, there are no long-term studies that evaluate efficacy or safety
- Severe carb restriction can be hard to adhere to long term and thus unsustainable
- Restrictive diets are more likely to result in micronutrient deficiencies

- There is evidence that a long-term negative impact on cardiac factors may outweigh any benefit in some individuals
- The benefits associated with Keto may be achieved using a less rigid and restrictive eating strategy

Low-Carb Diets

Low-carb diets have some of the same benefits as a Keto diet, though the specific benefits will depend on many factors such as the quality and quantity of carbs eaten as well as the overall quality of the diet. Both Atkins and Paleo are an example of a low-carb diet. In contrast to a very low-carb diet like Keto, which restricts carbs to ten to fifteen grams/day, a low-carb diet can range from 10 to 40 percent of total calories coming from carbs (50-200 grams if eating 2000 calories). That is quite a spread. Additionally, studies looking at low-carb diets are often based on diets where participants are eating as much as 50 percent of their calories from carbs.

Clearly, low-carb can look very different as not all low-carb diets follow the same rules. They are just all low-carb relative to current dietary patterns. For example, those who promote a Paleo lifestyle often recommend avoiding modern day grains, legumes, and night shades, a family of plants that include tomatoes, bell peppers, chili peppers, and potatoes.

A low-carb diet that focuses only on the macronutrient breakdown would be, at least in theory, easier to adopt and sustain than a strict Keto diet. Although, with Paleo, which is more restrictive in other regards, this is not necessarily true.

Due to a wide range of what constitutes low-carb, not all low-carb diets share the same benefits and/or potential risks since the content of the diet can vary considerably. As is true with Keto, the overall quality of the foods consumed may be even more important than the foods being avoided or restricted.

Pros

• May improve the overall quality of diet if whole, healthy foods are replacing processed carbs
  • May be better tolerated by those with insulin resistance
  • Depending on the specific low-carb diet, compared to a

strict Keto, may be easier to follow and adhere to over the short and long term

• May produce slightly more weight loss and better insulin sensitivity than low-fat diets, at least initially

Cons

• Adherence may be difficult, especially if the diet is relatively restrictive

• May lead to long-term micronutrient deficiencies, again depending on the restrictiveness of the diet

• The same benefits may be achieved through a less restrictive approach

The Mediterranean Diet

The Mediterranean diet is a relatively high-fat diet based on the traditional eating patterns of the Mediterranean.

It first became popular thanks to a scientist by the name of Ancel Keys, PhD, who conducted the Seven Countries study at the end of WWII. In the famous study, Keys compared the health outcomes of 13,000 men from Greece, Japan, Italy, the United States, Finland, the Neverlands, and former Yugoslavia.

He found that the men living in Crete had a significantly lower incidence of heart disease, which he attributed to their diet.

Since then, a number of published studies have established the benefits of this higher fat (roughly 40 percent), whole foods diet, including a lower risk of heart disease, diabetes, some cancers, and Alzheimer's.

A Mediterranean diet centers around vegetables, nuts, seeds, whole grains, beans, legumes, herbs, spices, and olive oil. Recommendations include eating fish and seafood at least twice a week, and poultry, eggs, cheese, yogurt, and wine in moderation. Sweets and other meats are consumed only occasionally.

Though there is no specific macronutrient breakdown, the Mediterranean diet tends to be higher fat, which may account for its high palatability and satiability.

Unrestrictive and easy to follow, the Mediterranean diet is a very sustainable eating strategy with studies linking it to good health outcomes.

Pros

- Benefits are well supported in the scientific literature
- Relatively non-restrictive
- Palatable and satiating
- Good compliance over the long term

- Can easily be followed while eating away from home

Cons

- Some people may not like fish, which is a big part of this way of eating and likely responsible for some of the observed health benefits
- People may overconsume things like bread, cheese, and wine which are associated with the diet but only intended to be eaten in moderation, while under-consuming vegetables, herbs, spices, beans, nuts, and seeds.

Fasting

Benjamin Franklin, an accomplished writer, scientist, inventor, diplomat, and statesman, once said, "The best of all medicines are resting and fasting." Rumi, the 13th century poet and scholar, claimed, "Fasting is the first principle of medicine; fast and see the strength of the spirit reveal itself." Plato, an Athenian philosopher, concurred and is credited with saying, "I fast for greater physical and mental efficiency." Plutarch, a Greek biographer, echoed the same sentiment when he said, "Instead of using medicine, better fast today." Finally, Philippus Paracelsus, one of the three fathers of Western Medicine, said, "Fasting is the greatest remedy—the physician from within."

And it was not just the great thinkers of the past who recognized the benefits of fasting. Most religions embrace some sort of fasting practice. Buddhist monks and nuns abstain from eating after their midday meal. Christians typically observe Ash Wednesday as a day for fasting and praying. During the month of Ramadan, Muslims fast from dawn to dusk. Finally, though not required, fasting is a customary practice among many Hindus.

And as we mentioned before, fasting was a treatment for epilepsy since as early as 500 B.C.

Clearly, our ancestors believed that fasting was a worthwhile practice with both health and spiritual benefits.

And today, fasting has recently emerged as a popular weight loss strategy. Specifically, a strategy coined intermittent fasting has gained a lot of attention. You may even be wondering if fasting is right for you.

In evaluating whether to adopt a regular and designated fasting period, it is important to define fasting as it is a term that can mean different things to different people.

At its core, fasting simply implies a period of food abstinence followed by a period of feeding. The duration of the fasting and feeding periods can vary from a daily extended overnight fast to several days of fasting. Also, what you can eat or drink during the fasting window may differ from practice to practice and from person to person. Fasting also implies nothing about what you consume during the eating window.

Just like low-carb diets may be quite different depending on the specific eating philosophy, so can fasting practices.

The most basic and popular form of fasting, often referred to as intermittent fasting, extends the overnight fast and limits the eating window to between twelve and four hours. People will often do a 12:12, 14:10, 16:8, 18:6, or 20:4. The first number represents the fasting period and the second represents the feeding period.

Another popular strategy is OMAD (one meal a day) as well as ADF (alternate day fasting). A 5:2 diet is not a true fast but involves eating what you normally would five days a week and keeping calories between 500-600 calories on the other two days.

Finally, a prolonged fast lasting from a few days to several days every month is a strategy employed by some hoping to reap the benefits of extended abstinence. Bone broth or small amounts of fat are sometimes allowed during a prolonged fast.

Generally speaking, the longer the fast, the greater the potential benefits, but also the greater the potential risks.

Shorter fasts are associated with improved insulin sensitivity, blood sugar control, gut health, and sleep. They can also assist with weight loss and weight maintenance.

Longer fasts promote all the above, but may also increase autophagy, a process in which the body cleans up dead or damaged cells, effectively slowing down the aging process.

There are minimal risks associated with shorter fasts (fasts that last less than twenty-four hours.) The risks of longer fasts tend to increase with fasting time and include headaches, dizziness, dehydration, and electrolyte imbalances. Though sometimes mild, these symptoms can be severe in some individuals.

Whether engaging in shorter or longer fasts, the benefits of the strategy reflect the behavior. Stop the behavior (switch the input) and you will experience a comparable change in output.

If you treat fasting like another diet (temporary change in eating patterns usually focused on calorie restriction and losing weight), any benefits you see are likely temporary. To continue to enjoy the benefits, fasting must become a lifestyle.

At least some benefits associated with fasting may be a function of calorie restriction, as limiting the eating window often lowers calorie consumption for obvious reasons. Still, other benefits appear linked directly to the actual fasting, meaning they go beyond any change in caloric consumption or even the quality of food eaten.

Autophagy

As mentioned above, one celebrated benefit of longer fasts is autophagy. *Auto* means self and *phagy* means to eat, therefore *autophagy* means to eat oneself.

Though an oversimplification, autophagy is a process by which the body cleans up and recycles dead or damaged cells. In this way, it may help to slow or minimize the normal effects of aging.

As we age, our body's ability to perform autophagy can decrease.

There are several ways to increase or stimulate autophagy that are beneficial to the body and body tissues. Fasting and/ or prolonged calorie restriction represent two such ways. Exercise is another.

Proponents of intermittent fasting like to claim that autophagy is one of its benefits. This may be true, at least in animal models. The problem is that while autophagy has anti-aging benefits, the role of intermittent fasting in promoting those benefits needs more evidence and clarification. There may also be a point where excessive autophagy contributes to poor outcomes. For example, autophagy may stimulate tumor cell growth, depending on a whole slew of other factors.

There seems to be an increasing consensus among experts that fasting can promote a beneficial type of autophagy. How often and how long you must fast to get the full benefit or even to get any benefit is still not clear. Finally, it is possible there could be a critical point at which fasting either does not work or works too well.

Pros

• Easily paired with another eating strategy
• High compliance especially with shorter duration fasts
• Has a long history with a growing body of support in the current literature for benefits and effectiveness
• Is simple to implement and follow
• Longer fasting periods may increase autophagy, a natural process associated with decreased aging

Cons

• May be inappropriate or risky for those on insulin or other meds requiring food
• More restrictive fasts can be dangerous if not done responsibly and with an awareness of the risks
• Longer period fasts may be harder to sustain over the long haul
• May not fit into your current lifestyle
• May not suit certain athletes in which a prolonged fasting strategy interferes with ideal fueling practices

Whole-Foods Plant-Based Diet

A whole-foods plant-based diet is exactly what its name implies: an eating strategy that focuses on eating primarily intact plant foods. These include beans, lentils, legumes, nuts, seeds, fruits, veggies, herbs, and spices. While animal products like eggs, milk, and meat are not absolutely excluded, they are eaten in lesser amounts relative to plants.

The scientific literature to date supports the benefits of a whole-foods plant-based diet that include better gut health, improved glucose control, and a decreased incidence of lifestyle diseases including heart disease, diabetes, high blood pressure, Alzheimer's, and many types of cancer.

There do not appear to be any major drawbacks to a whole-foods, plant-based diet, unless you decide to eliminate or severely restrict all animal products. Like other diets that severely restrict a food or groups of foods, micronutrient deficiencies are a concern. For example, vitamin B12 is primarily found in meat, while heme iron (iron from animal products) is much better absorbed than non-heme iron (iron found in plants.)

Pros

- Benefits well established and many
- Easy to follow
- Palatable and satiating
- Nonrestrictive and thus both adequate and safe

Cons

- While limiting processed foods is a good thing, it can be hard in today's food culture
- Micronutrient deficiencies may occur if animal products are significantly restricted or eliminated

Vegetarian (Pescetarian, Lacto Vegetarian, Ovo-Lacto Vegetarian, Ovo Vegetarian, Pollotarian, Flexitarian and Vegan)

All the above eating strategies are under the vegetarian umbrella and share one common theme: they avoid red meat and pork and restrict animal products to various degrees.

A **pescetarian** eats fish but restricts all other animal products. A **lacto-vegetarian** restricts all animal and animal byproducts except for dairy. The **ovo-lacto vegetarian** avoids meat but can consume eggs and dairy. An **ovo vegetarian** does not consume meat or dairy and dairy byproducts but eats eggs. A **pollotarian** restricts dairy, eggs, and most meat but will eat chicken. A **flexitarian** is someone who follows a plant-based diet but will occasionally eat animal or animal products and byproducts. Finally, a **vegan** avoids all animal and animal products, including dairy and eggs.

When talking about plant-based diets, the benefits of eating plants cannot be understated. They are loaded with micronutrients and phytonutrients known to promote health, protect against disease, and even treat or cure it.

That said, more restrictive vegetarian diets like vegan diets can be deficient in key nutrients such as B12.

Furthermore, just because something is a plant food does not mean it is a whole and intact food. Technically, high fructose corn syrup is a natural, plant-based food, albeit highly processed.

For this reason, eating any of the vegetarian diets and avoiding some or all animal products does not necessarily equate to healthy eating, especially if the plant foods you eat are highly refined ones. Just like with all the other eating strategies mentioned, the quality of what is eaten may be more important than what is being restricted. Not all vegetarian diets are healthy by default.

It is also worth noting that people may opt for a vegetarian diet based on principle, such as ethical considerations around the treatment of animals used in the production of meat, dairy, and eggs. For these individuals, the health benefits may be secondary to their concerns about animal welfare and/or the environment.

Whatever the case, it is important to understand the unique benefits and risks of any restrictive diet. The more restrictive, the greater the potential for deficiencies. And as stated previously, the quality of the food eaten, plant-based or not, matters.

Pros

• If choosing unrefined plant sources, the benefits are numerous and well established
• Are often better for the environment
• May align with your ethics around the treatment of animals
• Easy to follow
• Sustainable

Cons

• May not be a healthy diet if you choose refined and processed plant foods too often
• Could lead to micronutrient deficiencies, especially when exceptionally restrictive

80/20 Plan

Simply put, an 80/20 approach to eating involves eating whole or minimally processed foods 80 percent of the time while being more flexible with the other 20 percent. Like fasting, the 80/20 plan can be combined with other eating strategies.

The basic premise is sometimes good really is good enough. The emphasis is strictly on eating more intact whole foods while limiting rather than eliminating processed foods.

It is a simple strategy that is both flexible and easy to implement. By focusing on whole quality foods, quantity often takes care of itself. Additionally, allowing indulgences at an individual's discretion fosters compliance both in the short and long term. After all, the worst part of dieting is dieting.

Again, whole intact foods are those foods that you could grow or raise on the farm. These include fruits, vegetables, nuts, seeds, legumes, beans, lentils, herbs, spices, meat, eggs, and even dairy. Think farm to table. By consuming whole healthy foods most of the time, this way of eating promotes a diverse, inclusive diet that is nutritionally sound and easy to follow, whether dining at home or away.

Yet despite its simplicity, it is extremely effective, in part because it is so easy to follow and adopt long term. It is also easy to adapt to personal food preferences or food sensitivities and food allergies.

Many of the people I know with lean, strong, and healthy bodies follow an 80/20 strategy.

The one major drawback to this type of eating is it may not work well for someone who is struggling with food and/ or is confused about what constitutes a healthy food choice. Certain individuals may also need or prefer more guidance when it comes to portion control. Other than eating 80 percent intact whole foods, there are no rules, which might be great for someone who is already fit or knowledgeable about healthy eating patterns, but not as great for the novice who may be confused or have eating patterns that are out of control. Finally, those who are metabolically sick may benefit from not just whole foods but also a specific ratio of macronutrients, at least early on.

Pros

- Easy to follow
- Flexible
- High compliance
- Relatively unrestrictive
- Nutritionally diverse

Cons

- Provides minimal guidance
- May confuse a novice
- Unless paired with another strategy, may not always be the best choice for metabolically impaired individuals

Summary

There are many approaches to eating healthy that are not necessarily inclusive or exclusive. In the end, the best strategy is the one that not only supports your goals and desired outcomes, but that you can adhere to over the long haul. There is no one best strategy, but there is a strategy that is right for each of us. Part of the challenge is finding it, and part of finding it may mean experimenting to see what works and what does not.

Of course, we can tweak, switch, or refine a strategy as we go, but we cannot abandon it, not if we hope to sustain our gains. Again, consistency is key.

Just remember that there are no fixed rules. There is input and there is output, and different inputs can sometimes lead to the same output. On the other hand, the same input can sometimes result in different outputs for different people. This is because eating healthy can be as much an art as a science. We are all different. We have different genes, different bodies, different resources, different strengths, different tastes/preferences, and different weaknesses. For this reason, the science behind these various strategies should not necessarily dictate what we do. Instead, it should help to inform our decisions as we weigh the benefits and costs of different approaches against the backdrop of everything that makes us unique.

In the end, the best strategy is the one that works, and a multitude of factors may affect if and why something works, some obvious yet some not so obvious. In the first part of this book, I outlined strategies I found to be helpful. I know they work if consistently employed. But they certainly are not the only strategies or even the only effective strategies.

As much as people want to be told exactly what to do (what to eat, how much, and when), I cannot. I can give information and general guidance. I can educate about the potential risks and benefits. I can share what the current science says. I can suggest ways to work through barriers to change, but only the individual can figure what works for them because at the end of the day, only they must live with the choices they make.

FOOD SENSITIVITIES

At the age of ten, my daughter began experiencing regular bouts of diarrhea and vomiting. At first, we assumed it was a virus, but after several weeks of persistent symptoms, we suspected more. A trip to her doctor, who screened for all the usual suspects, produced negative results with one exception, a positive transglutaminase antibody test.

Her pediatrician was not particularly worried since all the other tests in that panel were normal but sent us to a gastroenterologist for further evaluation. And thus began my personal experience with a food intolerance.

After additional workups, doctors diagnosed my daughter with Celiac disease, an autoimmune disorder that causes an immune response to gluten, a protein found in wheat and barley.

Her diagnosis not only explained her recent bouts of gastrointestinal distress, but it also explained why, at the age of eight, she had to have four rotten teeth pulled and why, as an infant, she would projectile vomit anytime I attempted to give her baby cereal. Finally, it explained why she was small for her age and had a history of low vitamin D and iron.

Of course, this was only apparent in hindsight.

Interestingly, around the same time, my mother was having her own health issues. For some unknown reason, her blood volume was dropping. Within several months, she had received half a dozen blood transfusions.

While talking to her on the phone about my daughter's

diagnosis of Celiac disease, she casually mentioned that that was what one doctor thought she had. Like my daughter, she had tested positive for transglutaminase antibodies. However, because a follow-up biopsy of her small intestines failed to show microvilli blunting—the gold standard for the diagnosis of Celiac disease—my mother was told she did not have Celiac but had latent or potential Celiac (aka not Celiac or at least not yet). The doctors then sent her on her way, still with no answers.

I was not so quick to dismiss the possibility of Celiac. The surface area of the small intestines is huge. It is possible that there was microvilli blunting present that the testing simply missed. I also knew my mother's personal health history. From as far back as I could remember, my mother was plagued with gastrointestinal upset that included periods of unusual constipation to bouts of persistent diarrhea. She was constantly gassy and belching. She always kept a supply of tums, Pepto Bismol, stool softeners, and laxatives on hand. She also had been on Prilosec for much of her adult life to treat GERD (gastroesophageal reflux disease). To say this woman was a poster child for gastrointestinal upset is an understatement. A Celiac diagnosis not only seemed plausible, but it also seemed likely.

Celiac is genetic, which means my daughter got it from someone. So, I convinced my mom to go gluten-free. Within a few months, her mysterious blood loss, (the cause of which had yet to be identified) stopped, and her blood volume stabilized.

At the same time, all my daughter's symptoms also resolved on a gluten-free diet.

Coincidence?

I doubt it.

My mother has since repeatedly tested positive for transglutaminase antibodies, though never formally diagnosed with Celiac. She still eats a little gluten (at her age, giving up bread is a monumental undertaking), but she feels better when she does not.

Does she have true Celiac? Does it matter?

Whatever you want to call it, my mother, like my daughter, feels better when she avoids gluten.

True Celiac is an autoimmune disorder associated with a food intolerance. People with Celiac must avoid gluten, a protein found in wheat, or risk triggering an autoimmune event. It is not necessarily dose-dependent—as even tiny amounts can trigger the response—and you do not outgrow it. People who get it are genetically predisposed, though symptoms might not appear until later in life. The gold standard for a definitive diagnosis has always been microvilli blunting on biopsy of the small intestine.

For those who do not have the characteristic microvilli blunting but test positive on the blood tests and/or who feel better when avoiding gluten, we have created another label called *gluten sensitive*. Though not formally diagnosed with Celiac, gluten-sensitive individuals feel better when they do not eat gluten.

Finally, others may have a gluten or wheat allergy, which means the immune system sees these substances as an allergen and mounts a defensive response against them. Fortunately, the attack is not focused on healthy human cells, but on the allergen. Unfortunately, the reaction can range from mild and annoying to severe and life-threatening.

Whether intolerant, sensitive, or allergic, an individual may find that certain foods considered healthy, like whole wheat, may make them sick.

Furthermore, there are potential negative reactions to a whole spectrum of foods and/or the additives and preservatives used in their processing. From peanut allergies to lactose intolerance to wheat or gluten sensitivity. The possibilities are endless. Unfortunately, identifying a problem can sometimes be extremely difficult. Clinicians often misdiagnose or miss food sensitivities and treat the associated symptoms without ever understanding the underlying cause.

More recently, we have developed diagnostic tests such as blood tests that can aid doctors in making a definitive diagnosis. The problem is, like my mother, who suffered for years, affected individuals may not recognize something is wrong. They do not consider their symptoms as being unusual, abnormal, or severe enough to bring up with their doctor. And not all doctors are well informed about food sensitivities.

Common signs that you may have a food sensitivity include excessive and chronic bloating—particularly after meals—stomach cramps, diarrhea, constipation, indigestion, headache, nausea, vomiting, excessive and persistent congestion, and skin rashes.

Though experiencing these symptoms does not guarantee that you have a food sensitivity, they can all be warning signs suggesting you do, particularly if they are persistent or appear connected to a certain food or foods.

What should I do if I suspect I have a food sensitivity?

Increased awareness around food sensitivities has presented companies with another opportunity to capitalize on our health problems. As a result, there are currently several home test kits that claim to identify food sensitivities.

While this sounds great and there is no shortage of testimonials to tout their usefulness, I tend to be skeptical.

People who take these tests are often told they are sensitive to over a dozen common foods based on information garnered from a few drops of blood.

In response, they change their diet and report feeling better, thus in their minds confirming the accuracy of the test results. Only, it is very possible they feel better because they are eating better. Correlation is not causation.

The problem is that people may avoid foods they do not need to. We already know that diets that are excessively restrictive and/or eliminate certain foods are not only harder to sustain long term but can also contribute to nutrient deficiencies.

A better strategy would be to consult a nutritionist or functional medicine doctor who has experience in diagnosing and treating food sensitivities across the lifespan.

While it may be a little expensive, working one on one with a clinician who understands your health history and current medical status, including any food sensitivities, is the way to go. Any blood test needs to be correlated to your symptoms.

Of course, you can always try the home tests and experiment with elimination diets. Just keep in mind that identifying food sensitivities is often a tricky business.

Whatever you do, realize that just because a food or group of foods is considered healthy does not mean they will always be healthy for you. Finding a diet on which you thrive is often a process of trial and error, and it may sometimes require the help of a trained professional, which may or may not be your physician. Though physicians are becoming more aware of the role food sensitivities play in their patient's health, they may not always be the best person to help identify potential problems. So, when seeking professional advice, ask about a practitioner's experience with food sensitivities.

EXERCISE/ MOVEMENT STRATEGIES

W hen it comes to our health, exercise (aka regular, routine, and intentional movement) really is a magic pill. From the cardiopulmonary system to the musculoskeletal system to the endocrine system to the neurological system, there is not one organ that does not benefit from moving our bodies. Yet, exercise is often reduced to a means of creating a calorie deficit, a method to burn calories and lose weight. We forget that the real benefit of exercise lies not in its ability to increase our calorie expenditure but instead in its ability to fine-tune the machine and keep it in optimal working order. A healthy body is not only a fit body, but it will also support our efforts to achieve and maintain a healthy weight and level of leanness.

In the No Excuses Facebook group, people often ask what the best exercise is as if there were a single answer to that question. The reality is that *it depends*. The ideal mode/modes of exercise you choose should support your goals and may depend on several different variables such as your age, your current fitness level, your general health, your interests, your time constraints, and your access to various resources to name just a few. Ideally, you will include movement strategies that emphasize and develop all areas of fitness including flexibility, mobility, strength, muscular and cardiovascular endurance, balance, and coordination. Your movement strategy should also support your movement, fitness, and/or performance goals.

So, to help you better understand what type of movement that is best for you, in this chapter, I explore several popular modes of fitness/exercise.

Yoga

Though I took my first yoga class over three decades ago while an undergraduate at the University of Delaware to fulfill a PE requirement, it has only been in the last several years that I have practiced yoga with any purpose or regularity.

And I would like to highlight the word practice, as one of the best parts about yoga is you never master it. No matter how good you get, you can always tweak the pose to get even better.

On the flip side, you can also start a yoga practice at any age or level of fitness by modifying the poses to meet your body where it is at a particular moment in time.

When people think about yoga, they often think about flexibility and contorting their bodies into impossible poses. But it is so much more than that.

Yoga is the perfect blend of flexibility, mobility, balance and coordination, muscular strength, muscular endurance, and cardiovascular endurance. And that list only highlights the physical benefits. Ideally, a traditional yoga practice goes much deeper. Yoga, as a discipline, addresses the complete individual, physically, emotionally, and spiritually, as well as the individual's relationship with their surroundings.

Under the umbrella of yoga are several disciplines, including Vinyasa, Ashtanga, Hatha, Yin, Bikram, Kundalini, and Nidra.

These different disciplines all have slightly different emphases, but all of them are effective ways to build and improve fitness.

Vinyasa

Vinyasa links breath to movement. A typical Vinyasa class would involve a flow through classic poses with an emphasis on controlled breathing throughout the movement. Sometimes referred to as power yoga, Vinyasa can help develop strength, muscular endurance, flexibility and mobility, balance, and coordination. It even improves cardiovascular endurance as moving quickly between postures allows the heart rate to rise.

Ashtanga

Ashtanga is a type of Vinyasa practice that follows a set pattern of movement that does not change from class to class. In Ashtanga, students move through a series of poses independently. An instructor is available for correction only. The consistent content of an Ashtanga class may appeal to those who are new to yoga or comforted by the idea of a set routine. It also encourages mastery. Ashtanga offers many of the same benefits as Vinyasa. Additional benefits might include more mobility and flexibility as the poses may be held longer and the practice may be more involved.

Hatha

Hatha yoga is like Vinyasa and Ashtanga in that it emphasizes traditional yoga poses and breath, only in Hatha the poses are often held longer. This longer hold can be great for building muscular strength and endurance, balance, flexibility, and mobility.

Yin

Yin yoga also draws on traditional yoga poses only the emphasis is on a prolonged static hold, which allows for the stretching of non-contractile connective tissue such as ligaments and fascia. For this reason, Yin is more focused on developing flexibility and mobility, especially in the fascial system.

Bikram

Bikram yoga (also called hot yoga) involves performing the same twenty-six beginner poses in a hot and humid environment. While breathing is important, the real emphasis is on focus and concentration. The heat facilitates muscle extensibility, which allows participants to go deeper into poses than they might normally. It also taxes the cardiovascular system as your body works extra hard to dissipate heat. The format of the class, which covers twenty-six basic poses, also encourages mastery. In some respects, hot yoga could be considered HIIT training as the poses, which drive the heart rate up for short bursts, are followed by a resting pose/recovery. Bikram is good for improving cardiorespiratory fitness, muscular strength and endurance, balance, coordination, flexibility, and mobility. Its emphasis on breathwork and focus also adds a meditative quality to the practice.

Kundalini

Kundalini is a combination of breath, movement, meditation, and sound, which awakens your inner energy. Postures are held for prolonged periods and are accompanied by breathing exercises and a post-hold moment of internal reflection or meditation. Individuals who practice this type of yoga cite its spiritual nature in addition to its physical benefits.

Nidra

Yoga Nidra is a yogic sleep that transports participants to a place somewhere between wakefulness and sleep. A guided meditation, Nidra relieves stress and anxiety. Nidra can be performed independently or at the end of another practice/class. The goal is to develop a deeper connection between mind and body.

What is the best yoga practice for me?

Like most answers in this book, the answer is *it depends*. While most practices are safe for most people, there is no standard approach. For example, not everyone will enjoy or even tolerate the hot, humid temperatures of Bikram, at least not initially. Likewise, some might prefer the static and restorative nature of Yin to the continuous quicker paced flow of Vinyasa or vice versa. And still, others will enjoy a mix of different classes.

Pros

• Offers a number of class options that address all areas of fitness

• Emphasizes the whole person physically, emotionally, and spiritually

• Can address the needs of the advanced athlete and the novice because all practice can be modified to meet people where they are

• Accessible to people across the lifespan with modifications

• Offers variety

Cons

• May intimidate an individual based on their preconceptions about what yoga is

• Not all yoga classes or studios are created equal—they all have their own energy, personality, and vibe which may or may not mesh with you

• Not all classes will appeal to everyone, and some classes may better suit a specific individual, at least initially

Resistance Training

Resistance training includes any exercise in which you move your body against resistance, including free weights, kettlebells, bands, medicine balls, nautilus machines, sandbags, weighted vests, or even your body weight.

Resistance training can improve muscular strength and muscular endurance while helping to build and maintain lean body mass, including muscle and bone. When used as part of a high-intensity interval training program (which we will talk about in more depth later), it can also help to improve cardiorespiratory fitness.

The type, frequency, intensity, and time of resistance training will depend on your specific goals.

Muscular strength or power refers to the amount of weight you can lift for a single rep, whereas **muscular endurance** refers to how many times you can lift a specific load. Both are important. Finally, **muscular hypertrophy** refers to an increase in the size of the actual muscle.

As we age, we lose lean body mass, including muscle and bone. It's estimated that after the age of thirty, we can lose as much as 3 percent of our lean mass per year. Resistance training can prevent, slow down, and even reverse this loss of lean tissue.

For an exercise to qualify as resistance training, it must involve moving our bodies and joints against resistance. In the broadest sense, even walking is resistance training because our bodies and joints are working against the forces of gravity. As such, even low-impact activities can help to preserve muscle and bone. However, adding additional resistance such as dumbbells, kettlebells, and sandbags can up the ante and help to further strengthen our bones, our muscles, and the joints they move and support. It can also provide a way to shape and sculpt our bodies beyond a baseline starting point.

To get stronger and build muscle, you must overload the

muscle. Most people think of lifting weights when they think about building muscle. However, lifting an external weight like dumbbells is not the only effective strategy. For example, holding a yoga pose in which your muscles must work against the force of gravity to maintain a desired position can help to build and shape muscles while developing muscular strength and endurance, at least up to a certain point. Look at a dancer's glutes or a cycler's quads. A dancer must move their body against gravity in a way that requires a baseline muscular strength and muscular endurance. Likewise, a cycler must repeatedly push a pedal against resistance, a feat that also requires a certain amount of muscular strength and endurance.

Regardless of the movement, additional weight or resistance will further tax the muscle, leading to overload and a muscle that is stronger and/or has greater endurance. For example, increasing the weight used during a biceps curl can help to increase muscular strength, muscular endurance, and even hypertrophy in the specific group of muscles associated with that movement. Meanwhile, adding a weighted vest while engaged in an activity associated with cardiovascular conditioning like running not only improves cardiovascular fitness and function but also results in improved muscular strength and endurance of the skeletal muscles involved.

The heavier the load, the fewer reps you will be able to perform at any level of fitness because of the muscular strength and endurance it will require. If you are lifting weights and your primary goal is to get stronger at a particular task or movement like squatting, you must push yourself to work against heavier loads or loads at which you can perform one to six reps safely for three to four sets but few more. If your primary goal is to hypertrophy the muscle, then six to twelve reps are sufficient. Finally, if your primary goal is to develop muscular endurance, twelve plus reps will get it done.

And if you simply want a lean, strong, and healthy body, you may find moving against gravity in functional ways that support your chosen activities is all you need to succeed.

Whatever your mode of resistance, remember that muscle overload requires adequate recovery periods to be effective. The amount of recovery needed can depend on the type, intensity, and duration of the overload. The higher the resistance and the larger the overall load during a workout session, the longer the recovery may take. Although even this will depend on an individual's age, sex, starting fitness level, general health status, sleep, and nutrition.

Continuing to overload a muscle that has not fully recovered can result in injury. A good rule of thumb is to never train with extra resistance or in a way that overloads the muscle in question when still sore. On the other hand, a light jog or light stretching session can sometimes facilitate recovery.

In general, almost all exercise and movement helps to improve general muscle tone, muscle fitness, and performance. Increasing leanness by losing fat can also lead to a more muscular physique even in the absense of hypertrophy because it allows you to see the muscle. Gaining muscle mass and/or getting stronger may take more targeted and nuanced efforts that focuses on muscle overload.

What is the best way to incorporate resistance training into my fitness plan?

As described previously, there are a number of ways to incorporate resistance training into your fitness routine. What method you choose will depend on your goals, your current abilities, your personal preferences, and your fitness/ aesthetic goals. Those looking to put on substantial amounts of muscle weight will need to engage in exercises that overload the muscle adequately enough to stimulate muscle hypertrophy. Similarly, those who want to get stronger must lift heavier weights or at least weights that are heavy to them. In short, your methods should support your goals.

Pros

• Is one of the most effective ways to preserve and build lean body mass like muscle and bone

• Depending on your specific goals, can include many workout methods

• Again, depending on goals, body weight may achieve the desired outcome and may not require external equipment

Cons

• May require an external source of resistance

• Depending on goals, may require a more nuanced and specialized approach

• Could feel intimidating especially for those who are older and/or considered frailer

Cardiorespiratory Fitness Training (Steady-State)

Steady-state cardio includes low, moderate, and sometimes even higher intensity activities like biking, jogging, running, or swimming. While challenged, you are not so challenged that you cannot maintain a steady pace for a prolonged duration.

Cardiovascular exercise requires the use of large muscles like the quads. These muscles require oxygen which must be delivered via the lungs and heart. During cardio, your breathing rate increases as the body attempts to provide the oxygen necessary to convert stored calories into a usable form of energy. Heart rate also increases to get this oxygen to its destination. If you can meet your energy needs via an oxygen-mediated pathway, an activity is considered **aerobic** (or in the presence of oxygen.)

The heart is also a muscle and stressing it via steady-state training can improve its function. Likewise, the lungs get better at doing their job via an increase in lung capacity which is their ability to fill with air and take in more oxygen. There are other positive adaptations as well. In response to cardiovascular exercise, your body gets better at transporting oxygen. It also increases the number of mitochondria in various cells, which are cellular structures where oxygen is used to produce cellular energy in the form of ATP. The benefits of steady-state cardio correlate to the intensity at which you are working. The harder you work, the greater the benefits. The heart is a muscle and any activity that stresses it can lead to improved function.

Pros

• Because steady-state cardio often involves activities performed at a low to moderate intensity, it is safe for most fitness levels
• Many people enjoy the longer duration repetitive moves associated with running, swimming, cycling etcetera
• Steady-state promotes cardiorespiratory fitness and general well-being relative to the intensity

Cons

• Often requires significant time investment to achieve desired goals
• May not result in improved cardiorespiratory fitness beyond a specific baseline
• May be able to get the same or even superior benefits from alternatives like High-Intensity Interval Training in a fraction of the time

High-Intensity Interval Training

As the name implies, high-intensity interval training—HIIT for short—is a training strategy that incorporates bouts of extremely high intensities (think hard to breathe or sustain moves) with bouts of lower and sometimes even low-intensity movement.

The idea is to work at an unsustainable intensity for short bursts, often less than a minute, and then to engage in a recovery phase. This cycle is repeated anywhere from ten to thirty minutes.

HIIT has recently become immensely popular because it not only offers the traditional benefits of steady-state cardio training but also delivers those benefits in a fraction of the time. This is huge when you consider lack of time is a common excuse for not exercising.

In his book *The One Minute Workout*, researcher Martin Gibala reveals the science behind HIIT and explains why it can be such a great strategy, particularly for those who have time constraints. He even shares his one-minute workout. Though it takes ten minutes to complete, Gibala's one-minute workout incorporates three twenty-second rounds of super high-intensity moves (thus the one-minute name) with a warm-up, cool-down, and two two-minute recoveries.

According to Gibala, not only are total calories comparable to a much longer session of steady state at a moderate intensity thanks to EPOC (excess post-exercise oxygen consumption), there are cellular changes that support improved cardiorespiratory fitness that are not only equal to steady state but exceed it.

Excuses be gone!

Who does not have at least ten minutes a day?

There are many ways to create and take part in HIIT. Though the high-intensity portion of the workout can vary, it needs to be hard. Think short bursts or sprints that last 10-20 seconds periodically performed during a walk or light jog. Pushing ourselves beyond our comfort zone strengthens us and improves fitness.

A drawback of HIIT is that it requires higher-intensity moves. For example, thirty seconds of strict burpees would challenge even the fittest among us, but those types of high-intensity moves are not for everyone.

Other examples of high-intensity moves include sprinting, plyometrics like box jumps, and heavy lifts that approach a person's one-rep max. A lower-impact option would include cycling on an incline or at an extremely high speed. Any activity that requires an intensity that cannot be sustained for more than a couple of minutes would be classified as high intensity for that individual.

Most people can usually find a safe way to challenge themselves, it may just take extra thought or even coaching from a fitness professional who understands an exerciser's unique needs and abilities.

Benefits associated with HIIT include increased explosiveness, improved cardiorespiratory fitness, autophagy, and improved metabolic function beyond what one might achieve with steady-state alone. Thus, incorporating HIIT sessions into your training regimen can offer substantial health and performance benefits. And most importantly, it requires a lower time investment.

Pros

• Can provide benefits beyond steady-state in a fraction of the time
• Can be a great option for those looking to switch things up or to get the benefits of resistance training and cardio training simultaneously

Cons

• Working at higher intensities may not be safe or realistic for all individuals
• Working at high intensities is often uncomfortable and forces us to temporarily push ourselves to a level of discomfort that is unattractive to some

ANATOMY AND PHYSIOLOGY 101: GAINING HEALTH VS LOSING WEIGHT

We often use words like healthy and thin interchangeably, even though they are not mutually inclusive or exclusive. For example, just because a behavior supports weight loss or thinness does not mean it is healthy or always supports health. Yet, people continue to employ weight loss-centered rather than health-centered strategies when trying to get leaner, not realizing that good health is a prerequisite to reaching and maintaining a lean, strong, and healthy body over the long haul.

A healthy body is one in which all the body systems work together to keep the machine functioning well. A healthy immune system keeps us from getting sick. A healthy endocrine system regulates the sleep-wake cycle, hunger, satiety, and a whole slew of other important bodily functions via hormones, while a healthy cardiovascular, musculoskeletal, and neurological system allows us to participate in the many adventures of life without significant limitation. Though overweight and obesity are independent risk factors for chronic disease, and losing weight can have a positive impact on health regardless of how we lose it, simply limiting calories and creating calorie deficits does not always support our long-term health. Prolonged calorie deficits coupled with restrictive diets that focus primarily on calories and/or macros and sweat sessions focused exclusively on calories burned often miss the mark when it comes to promoting health over the life span. And a healthy body will radiate health externally via radiant skin, toned muscles, healthy joints, and an aesthetically pleasing and lean body. A healthy body that is working properly supports all the systems designed to keep us not only healthy but also at a healthy weight.

In short, if health is not your primary goal, then it should be.

In this section, I have outlined the various body systems, what they do, and describe how—when working properly— they support a lean, strong, and healthy body. My goal is to illustrate why it is not simply about calories, calorie deficits, or even losing weight. The best way to obtain the body of your dreams is to focus on building a lean, strong, and healthy body with an emphasis on healthy by adopting healthy behaviors that not only support leanness or weight loss but that support optimal function of each body system.

Musculoskeletal System

The musculoskeletal system includes bones, ligaments, and fascia (non-contractile tissue that provides structure) as well as muscles and tendons (contractile units that provide a means for locomotion and movement).

Bones

Like all other structures in the body, bone is living tissue that requires ongoing maintenance and nourishment. With a strong, rigid outer layer of compact bone called cortical bone and a lighter weight, spongy matrix called cancellous or trabecular bone, our bones cannot only withstand tremendous force, but they are also relatively lightweight.

Bones not only provide structure, but they also protect internal organs like the heart, lungs, and brain. They can serve as reservoirs for fat and minerals, and they produce hormones and blood cells.

We are born with about 300 bones, some of which are made of cartilage that will eventually harden. As we age, bones fuse so that we end up with 206 bones. Early in life, our bones can grow, a process that happens at the epiphyseal plates. Also known as growth plates, the bone epiphysis is composed of hyaline cartilage and is at the ends of long bones. Bones can continue to grow until the epiphyseal plate closes around the end of puberty.

Bone density refers to the amount of bone minerals in our bones. Most bone density is determined around the adolescent years. After this point, bones tend to lose density although the rate and amount of loss will depend on genetics, activity, and nutrition among other things.

Bones are living tissue with regular tissue turnover. Bone resorption refers to the ability of the body to replace old bone with new bone.

When we lose bone over the course of our lives, we

can develop a condition called osteopenia (initial stages of osteoporosis) or full-blown osteoporosis (a serious condition in which the bones become brittle and fragile).

Many people already know that a sufficient source of nutrients like calcium and vitamin D play a significant role in bone health over the lifecycle. However, other key nutrients include vitamin K, silicon, boron, magnesium, zinc, manganese, and copper. As a result, poor or inadequate nutrition can affect bone health.

The potential detrimental impact of other nutrients or substances like high-protein diets or other high-acid foods on bone health is complex and still poorly understood.

Regular exercise, particularly those that involve weight bearing or resistance, helps to form and maintain strong, healthy bones as we age.

Likewise, as we discussed earlier under the hormone section, low body fat in women that results in amenorrhea— an irregular or absent menstrual cycle—causes bone mineral loss. While completing my degree in Nutritional Sciences at the University of Delaware, the Nutrition and Dietetics department was studying the University's elite female ice skating team. These young women were the epitome of fitness on the outside but had the bones of eighty-year-old women thanks to their extremely low body fat.

General Recommendations for Bone Health

Regular exercise (especially weight-bearing and resistance exercise) combined with a plant-based diet high in fruits and veggies, low in processed foods, and that contains adequate sources of calcium and vitamin D promotes strong, healthy bones throughout the lifespan.

Ligaments

Ligaments are thick bands of fibrous connective tissue that attach bones to other bones and provide stability for joints (the area where two bones meet).

Ligamentous laxity varies from person to person and is influenced by genetics. Natural variation in ligamentous laxity explains why some individuals (those with looser ligaments) are good dancers or gymnasts and others (those with stiffer ligaments) are successful powerlifters and linebackers. In addition to genetics, training techniques, sport demands, and injury can all overstretch ligaments, contributing to an increase in ligamentous laxity. An overstretched, extremely lax, or injured ligament often results in joint hypermobility and even instability, while a medical condition like Ehlers-Danlos can result in severe laxity of the ligaments and joints, leading to chronic pain and frequent subluxation or dislocation culminating in excessive wear and tear on the joints.

Exercise that applies stress through the ligament without overloading it to the point of tissue deformation and injury can lead to stronger, healthier ligaments. Adequate nutrition and hydration also play a role.

If injured, some ligaments will heal while others will not. Those that do not heal may need to undergo surgical reconstruction to ensure a stable joint. This reconstruction may use a tendon or piece of ligament from your own body or one from a cadaver. For those ligaments that can heal, it is important to note that the resultant ligament is often weaker, leading to increased joint laxity and joint wear and tear that can culminate in arthritis and other joint problems. Gentle and modified movements during the healing phase, as opposed to prolonged immobilization, can improve the healing outcome.

A healthy joint will have a balance between mobility and stability. For those with naturally lax ligaments, an increased emphasis on strengthening the surrounding musculature is important. On the other hand, those with stiffer ligaments may need to spend more time actively working on flexibility and mobility.

General Recommendations for Ligamentous Health

Regular exercise, proper training techniques that protect normal joint function, and proper nutrition and hydration are important in maintaining healthy ligaments. Those who have excessive joint laxity because of injury, genetics, or a disease like Ehlers-Danlos may need to spend more time strengthening the muscles around that joint to help compensate. On the other hand, those with stiffer ligaments may need to spend more time focusing on activities that promote joint mobility and flexibility. Likewise, an injured ligament may never regain its original tensile strength, or it may require surgical reconstruction. Gentle movement and stress applied early after an injury produces better outcomes but should be catered to the injury.

Fascia

Fascia is a fibrous connective tissue made up of bundles of collagen that supports, joins, separates, and compartmentalizes the entire body. It also has a nerve supply, which means it receives and transmits valuable input from the muscles and organs to the spinal cord and brain.

What many of us think of as muscle tightness may instead reflect restrictions in the fascia, a structure designed to move, stretch, and reduce friction between adjacent structures but that can become dehydrated, scarred, and sticky secondary to injury, surgery, chronic postures (such as sitting hunched at a computer for eight hours a day), repetitive movements (such as key board typing or assembly line tasks), immobilization, and inactivity.

When fascia becomes tight or unable to function properly, it can cause pain and stiffness. In addition, when you apply a stretch to inflexible fascia, it can compress surrounding muscles, causing the development of painful knots and/or trigger points. Many of the conditions I treat as a physical therapist in the clinic have a fascial component.

Low-load, prolonged stretches like those employed in Yin yoga are an effective way to stretch tight fascia. Heat, movement, shorter duration stretches, and massage/manual therapy techniques also help.

General Recommendations for Fascial Health

An active and healthy lifestyle that includes regular exercise, proper nutrition, and hydration, while limiting chronic repetitive stresses and prolonged poor postures is the best way to keep fascia healthy. Heat, stretching (especially low-load prolonged stretches), massage, soft tissue mobilization, and early initiation of modified movement soon after injury or surgery can promote and/or restore normal fascia function.

Muscle

Muscle is contractile tissue that can shorten and lengthen. In the case of skeletal muscle, it culminates in a tendon made of non-contractile tissue that inserts into the bone. We have three types of muscle: cardiac, smooth, and skeletal.

Cardiac Muscle

Cardiac muscle is an involuntary, specialized, striated muscle found only in the heart. It is dubbed involuntary because the contraction of cardiac muscle is not under volitional control but controlled by portions of the brainstem and the hypothalamus.

Smooth Muscle

Smooth muscle—also known as visceral muscle—is an involuntary, non-striated muscle controlled by the autonomic nervous system. Examples of smooth muscle can be found in blood vessels, the intestinal tract, the stomach, the lungs, and other organs.

Skeletal Muscle

Skeletal muscle is voluntary contractile muscle, meaning we can actively control its function. It is also striated and attaches to bones via tendons. Innervated by nerves, skeletal muscle is responsible for creating and/or resisting movement about a joint.

Skeletal muscle is composed of muscle fiber bundles. Each muscle fiber is composed of the myofilaments **actin** and **myosin**. It is the organization of these myofilaments that give skeletal muscle its striated appearance and its ability to contract. A **sarcomere** represents one contractile unit within a muscle and each muscle has many sarcomeres. The **sliding filament theory** explains the mechanism by which skeletal muscle contracts. In short, actin and myosin filaments slide over each other bringing the ends of the sarcomere closer together, shortening the individual sarcomeres, and causing the muscle to contract.

Other Classifications

Muscle fibers are further classified as slow oxidative, fast glycolytic, or fast oxidative. **Slow oxidative** fibers contract slowly and use aerobic (in the presence of oxygen) pathways to provide energy as ATP. **Fast glycolytic** fibers contract quickly and depend exclusively on anaerobic (in the absence of oxygen) pathways. **Fast oxidative** fibers contract quickly and depend on aerobic (in the presence of oxygen) pathways for ATP. However, unlike slow oxidative fibers, they can switch to anaerobic (in the absence of oxygen) pathways when necessary.

Genetics heavily influence the proportion of each fiber type in a muscle. Individuals with a higher proportion of fast glycolytic fibers may have a small though real advantage when it comes to the explosiveness associated with sprinting or powerlifting while those with a higher proportion of slow oxidative fibers may make better endurance athletes.

Training can also play a factor since fast oxidative fibers can be conditioned to perform like slow oxidative or fast glycolytic fibers.

General Recommendations for Muscle Health

Both cardiac muscle and skeletal muscle can benefit from training and proper nutrition. Because the heart is a muscle that contracts, it can become stronger when periodically stressed through activities like steady-state cardio and high-intensity interval training. Any exercise or activity that results in an elevated heart rate can improve heart muscle function. Likewise, skeletal muscle can gain strength, size, and endurance when trained properly. Furthermore, exercise can also slow down the rate of muscle loss that we typically experience as we age, while improving the health, flexibility, resiliency, and function of our muscles, tendons, fascia, and ligaments. Finally, nutrition can also affect muscle health, as it provides the building blocks for all body tissues. And don't forget that while eating adequate protein in the diet is important for overall health as we discussed in the macronutrient chapter, simply increasing protein in the diet does not necessarily lead to an increase in muscle size or overall body muscle mass.

Exercise that overloads a muscle requires adequate recovery. Failure to adequately rest a muscle after significant overloading can contribute to tendinitis, bursitis, and even muscle tears and stress fractures.

Cardiorespiratory System

The cardiorespiratory system includes the heart, lungs, and blood vessels that carry both oxygenated and deoxygenated blood, important nutrients, hormones, and waste products throughout the body. Diseases of the heart and lungs are major contributors to morbidity and mortality worldwide.

Heart

As we learned previously, the heart is made of involuntary, striated contractile muscle. It is best described as an active pump designed to circulate blood throughout the body.

Lungs

The lungs are inflatable sacs responsible for inhaling air filled with oxygen and exhaling carbon dioxide. Our cells need oxygen, which is an important part of the chemical reactions necessary to access energy from the foods we eat.

Blood Vessels

Arteries are vessels that carry oxygenated blood and nutrients to our tissues via an active pumping system, aka the heart. **Veins** carry the deoxygenated blood along with waste products away from those same tissues, a process that is aided by muscle contraction and a series of valves.

We breathe air into our lungs where it is absorbed into the bloodstream. The arterial system pumps the oxygenated blood out to the rest of the body. The venous system, or veins, will transport the deoxygenated blood back to the heart and eventually the lungs where the process happens all over again.

Cardiovascular exercises like running, biking, and swimming are not simply a way to burn calories. These exercises, if done at a sufficient intensity, tax the cardiorespiratory system, which improves its fitness and function.

Our heart is a muscle that can get stronger, pumping out more blood with each stroke. But the body also adapts in other ways. In response to exercise that increases our heart rate, the number of mitochondria in our cells increases. **Mitochondria** are cellular powerhouses that derive energy from the foods we eat which is then used to fuel our cells. Furthermore, our lung capacity (our ability to take in air) increases. Finally, our ability to transport oxygen increases thanks to increases in hemoglobin and red cell mass along with the number of capillaries feeding our tissues.

Besides exercise, the foods we eat can also have an impact on the cardiorespiratory system. Diets high in processed foods like refined grains, meats, and oils have been linked to chronic systemic inflammation. This chronic inflammation (which is different from the acute inflammation observed with an injury like an ankle sprain) can lead to the stiffening of the arteries and the buildup of plaque inside the vessel wall. When this happens, the heart must work harder to get blood with its precious nutrients to our cells. Over time, this can cause a diseased and enlarged heart. Furthermore, if the narrowing of the vessel is significant enough, it can cause a blockage, culminating in a heart attack or a stroke.

It is worth taking a moment to differentiate between low-level, chronic systemic inflammation and the acute inflammatory response. The latter is part of the healing process while the former is a major contributor to lifestyle diseases. When we have an injury, the body responds by sending cells to the site of injury to clean up dead and injured cells and to lay down new, healthy tissues. Though this type of inflammation can become severe and lead to pain and stiffness, it is good and essential for healing to occur. On the other hand, low-level chronic systemic inflammation is often caused by repeated stress to the body and is the result of poor diet, inadequate exercise and sleep, and chronic stress. This type of inflammation is bad and contributes to all chronic lifestyle diseases.

For these reasons, cardiorespiratory fitness not only affects our ability to engage in life but is also a major contributing factor to death in most developed countries.

General Recommendations for Cardiorespiratory System Health

Eating a diet high in whole intact foods, particularly healthy plant foods (an excellent source of fiber), while also limiting refined foods helps to prevent chronic systemic inflammation while promoting the health of all organ systems, including the cardiorespiratory system.

Also, regularly taking part in exercises that tax the cardiorespiratory system, like steady-state cardio or high-intensity interval training, will go a long way toward ensuring optimal function of the heart and lungs. Just thirty minutes of cumulative (not necessarily continuous) low-to-moderate intensity activity at least five days a week is enough to lower an individual's risk of most chronic lifestyle diseases, including those that affect the heart and lungs. Hopefully you can now appreciate why the purpose of cardio exercise should not be solely to burn calories but instead to improve fitness of the the cardiorespiratory system.

Endocrine System

The endocrine system includes several organs: the pancreas, the pineal gland, the pituitary, the thyroid, the ovaries, the testis, and the adrenal gland. Its primary role is the regulation of body systems via hormones. It plays an active role in growth and development, metabolism, sleep, emotions, and mood, as well as overseeing homeostatic feedback loops.

Both blood pressure and blood sugar are carefully controlled by the endocrine system and the sensitive feedback loops designed to keep our bodies working properly even as internal and external forces change.

Both exercise and diet can affect the endocrine system. For example, diets high in processed and refined foods are associated with conditions like metabolic syndrome and type

2 diabetes, both characterized by insulin resistance. If you recall, insulin is an important hormone essential to dealing with incoming calories. It is also a pro-fat anabolic hormone that inhibits the release of glucagon and prevents the mobilization of stored calories like fat. On the other hand, diets high in whole foods not only prevent these diseases of the endocrine system, but they may also help to reverse them. Our eating habits can also affect the powerful hunger and satiety hormones leptin and ghrelin, both of which may be implicated in appetite, hunger, food consumption, weight gain, and difficulty losing weight. Finally, healthy, whole foods play a role in normalizing and optimizing sex hormones like estrogen and progesterone.

Another link between diet and the endocrine system involves our gut. Processed foods like those commonly eaten as part of the SAD diet (Standard American Diet) are low in fiber and thus may contribute to a leaky gut. Though we will discuss leaky gut in more detail when we discuss the digestive system, just know that it can affect the endocrine system via autoimmunity, which targets glands like the thyroid or organs like the pancreas.

Exercise, too, has been shown to have both an immediate and long-term positive influence over endocrine function. For example, a single bout of exercise can improve insulin sensitivity. And while many forms of exercise result in a temporary increase in cortisol levels, regular activity that challenges us are associated with overall lower levels of cortisol.

Exercise and diet can also directly and indirectly affect sleep. Insufficient and/or poor-quality sleep affects our hormones. Eating or drinking (especially alcohol or caffeinated beverages) too close to bedtime has been found to disrupt sleep. This can negatively affect both cortisol levels and insulin sensitivity, thus also impacting hunger, cravings, and satiety.

General Recommendations for Endocrine System Health

Eating a diet high in fiber-rich, whole, intact plant foods while limiting processed food is essential to promote healthy body systems but especially of the endocrine system, which is intimately related to metabolism and the way our body processes, mobilizes, and utilizes the calories we eat. Exercise, too, plays a key role in keeping the endocrine system working properly.

Finally, adequate sleep and stress management can be detrimental to the endocrine system which must continuously respond to stressors in our environment.

Digestive System

Digestion is a complex process that starts in the mouth with the mechanical action of chewing and mixing food with saliva and that ends with the excretion of waste and waste byproducts. It includes a multitude of structures, including the esophagus, the pharynx, the stomach, the small intestines, the large intestines, and the rectum. It also depends on accessory organs like the pancreas, liver, and gallbladder as well as glands, such as the salivary glands.

Food enters the mouth where it is chewed and mixed with saliva. Once swallowed, it enters the stomach, where it is further digested by stomach acids and a churning motion. This initial process produces a substance known as chyme. This is also where the chemical breakdown of proteins, carbs, and fats begins. Here in the stomach, food particles are broken down into even smaller pieces before entering the small intestines where much of the absorption of nutrients will take place.

Once in the small intestines, chyme is mixed with more digestive juices and slowly propelled onward. The small intestines are covered with tiny finger-like projections called microvilli that significantly increase its surface area and allow for maximal absorption of digested fats, proteins, and carbs. It also allows the absorption of vitamins, minerals, and phytonutrients.

Accessory organs like the liver produce bile salts, which aid in the digestion of fats, while the gallbladder stores, concentrates, and releases bile. Finally, the pancreas produces digestive enzymes.

Anything not absorbed in the small intestines enters the large intestines. Here, excess water and residual electrolytes and vitamins are reabsorbed. What remains is concentrated and propelled toward the rectum where it is stored until it can be excreted.

The foods we eat have a significant impact on the digestive system, including the small and large intestines.

As mentioned previously, the intestinal lining covers a large amount of surface area thanks to its finger-like projections, the microvilli. Because absorption occurs in the small intestines, its lining is selectively semipermeable to the digested macronutrients and micronutrients. However, permeability can be excessive thanks to unhealthy dietary habits that cause a condition known as **leaky gut**. A leaky gut loses some of its selectivity which means it allows things to pass that should not. This increased permeability can permit toxins, bugs, and even partially digested food to leak into the bloodstream. Diseases including Celiac, Crohn's, and irritable bowel syndrome have all been linked to leaky gut. There is also mounting evidence that a leaky gut may be implicated in other autoimmune disorders like lupus, type I diabetes, multiple sclerosis, fibromyalgia, chronic fatigue syndrome, and even skin conditions like acne.

Though certain individuals may be genetically predisposed to a leaky gut, lifestyle can play a key role. For example, as we mentioned earlier, the SAD diet, an acronym for the Standard American Diet, is high in sugar and processed foods and low in fiber and is associated with gut inflammation. The unhealthy, processed foods we eat can affect the bacteria that grow and thrive in the intestinal tract, resulting in an undesirable microbiome composition. This altered microbiome weakens the chemical bonds that make up the intestinal wall. Excess alcohol, late-night eating ,and too many hours of the day spent chowing down may also be factors as they interfere with necessary gut maintenance.

Though not as well understood, regular exercise and adequate sleep both promote gut health while stress can harm it.

Regarding exercise, even low-intensity movement can increase gut motility, thus decreasing contact time with various pathogens. It has also been shown to reverse negative changes associated with a high-fat diet and a sedentary lifestyle. Several studies suggest different modes of exercise may improve the intestinal microflora both from a qualitative and quantitative standpoint independent of diet. In short, exercise has been shown to not only increase the diversity of microflora but also the composition of microflora which promotes health and fights disease.

General Recommendations for Digestive System Health

Eating a diet high in whole, intact plant foods and high in fiber supports a diverse and healthy microbiome. This is because the good bugs that live in our gut eat the fiber we cannot digest. Interestingly, as we pointed out earlier, only about one in ten Americans get the recommended daily serving of fiber (some estimates are as low as one in twenty), even as many stress about getting enough protein. Coincidentally, only one in ten Americans also get the minimum recommended daily servings of fruits and veggies.

Though probiotics (those important microbes) and prebiotics (the food they eat) are often sold in supplement form, there is mounting evidence that supplementing alone does not cultivate a healthy gut microbe diversity, especially in the absence of a diet that supports a healthy microbiome. This is because our behaviors either promote or inhibit the growth of a healthy microbiome. Simply taking a pill does nothing to provide an internal environment in which a healthy gut microbiome can flourish.

Regular exercise, adequate sleep, and stress management have all been linked to the health of our microbiome, too.

The Immune System

The immune system is comprised of bone marrow, the thymus, the spleen, the tonsils, the lymphatic system, and the adenoids. Its primary role is to protect us from infection and to help heal via an inflammatory response.

When our immune system is strong and healthy, our bodies can fight off many infections caused by viruses, bacteria, and fungi. However, when our immune system is compromised, it can have catastrophic consequences for our health.

For example, in the most recent COVID-19 pandemic, data has shown that in those with a compromised immune system (such as the elderly) or those with chronic lifestyle diseases associated with systemic inflammation (such as type 2 diabetes, heart disease, or high blood pressure) infection with COVID is more likely to result in severe symptoms, hospitalization, ventilation, and even death secondary to complications.

Having a healthy immune system plays a critical role in not only surviving but also thriving. Unfortunately, many people routinely engage in behaviors that actually suppress and/or compromise their immune system function. Pro-inflammatory diets high in processed foods such as the Standard American Diet, inadequate sleep, lack of regular exercise, and poorly managed stress have all been linked to an impaired immune system. A compromised immune system might not only affect our body's ability to fight off communicable diseases caused by viruses and bacteria, but it also increases our risk of developing non-communicable diseases (lifestyle diseases) like type 2 diabetes, cardiovascular disease, high blood pressure, cancer, and even Alzheimer's. For example, in 2020, heart disease, cancer, and diabetes combined resulted in 1.4 million American deaths. The presence of a non-communicable disease also significantly impacted the mortality and morbidity associated with COVID.

Diet, specifically, has been linked to autoimmunity, a condition in which our immune system attacks our own cells. Though there is often a genetic predisposition for autoimmune diseases, environmental triggers that include our lifestyle choices play a role. The microbiome is a major player when it comes to autoimmunity, and as we learned previously, what we eat, how much we move and sleep, combined with the amount of stress in our life may all influence the gut flora.

General Recommendations for Immune System Health

Like the systems mentioned before it, promoting the health of the immune system includes eating a mostly whole-foods diet high in fiber-rich plant foods, moving in ways that challenge our body but still feel good, getting sufficient restorative sleep, and managing excess stress.

It is worth noting that many tactics employed for weight loss can harm rather than help the immune system function because of the extreme stress they place on the body. Prolonged calorie restriction (especially when care is not taken to ensure quality calories are being consumed) paired with extreme workouts which focus primarily on calorie deficits and often without adequate recovery cannot only cause injury, it potentially weakens the immune system. This is a perfect example of how an effective weight loss strategy (at least in the short term) is not necessarily consistent with better health.

The Nervous System

The nervous system is often broken down into two primary systems: the **central nervous system** or the CNS and the **peripheral nervous system** or the PNS.

The CNS includes the brain, the brain stem, and the spinal cord, while the PNS includes the peripheral nerves that travel throughout the entire body.

Organs like our eyes, ears, and skin collect external information that is transmitted to the CNS via peripheral nerves. Once in the CNS, the information is processed and acted upon.

Executive orders are carried to organs, muscles, and other structures via the nerves that innervate them.

Just like all other organs and organ systems, the nervous system is both directly and indirectly impacted by lifestyle choices, including nutrition, exercise, sleep, and stress.

Concerning nutrition, vitamin deficiencies—particularly those that involve the B vitamins—can affect nerve health and nerve function directly.

But nutrition can also impact the nervous system indirectly via the microbes that live in our gut as they communicate with the brain using what is known as the gut-brain axis. The trillion bugs housed in our gut both produce and consume neurotransmitters, chemicals that assist with nerve and brain function.[27]

Dietary strategies, such as fasting and Keto, that result in ketosis are neuroprotective, at least in a handful of animal models.[28] Whether via an increase in autophagy or some other mechanism, ketosis may play a role in keeping the brain young while decreasing the risks of brain diseases like Parkinson's and Alzheimer's. Analogously, a diet high in fruits and veggies that provides powerful antioxidants may also help to prevent diseases of the CNS and PNS by preventing oxidative damage to the various structures.

Exercise can also help to improve the health and function of the nervous system. For example, exercise can improve blood flow to various organs, including the brain. It is also associated with improved blood sugar control. Chronic hyperglycemia (too much sugar in the blood) can cause damage to the blood vessels that support all our organs, contributing to diseases and impaired function. It can also damage the nerves.

Likewise, exercise is known to improve balance responses in both the young and old alike by stimulating the peripheral nervous system and the central nervous system in equal measure. Studies have shown that regular exercise not only decreases the risks of developing brain diseases like dementia, Alzheimer's, and Parkinson's, but it can also slow down the progression and help ease or mitigate the symptoms.

For instance, a review of eleven studies looking at the impact of a regular yoga practice on the brain found that it had a positive impact on cerebral blood flow and several brain functions.[29] Yoga also reduces anxiety and other maladies associated with mental health.

The spinal cord and the peripheral nerves are also affected by the health of the spinal column, including the muscles, joints, tissues, and other structures involved in its function. The health of these structures can be significantly affected by exercise, movement, and lack of movement.

Sleep is another major player in the health of our nervous system. As we have already learned, quality of sleep or lack of sleep can negatively affect hormones like cortisol, ghrelin, and insulin, which impact our CNS and PNS. A poor night's sleep can affect concentration, memory, focus, and even our reflexes. Inadequate sleep has also been linked to the buildup of the harmful plaques observed in Alzheimer's. In at least one study, a single night of poor sleep was associated with an increase in beta-amyloid, a protein in the brain associated with impaired brain function and Alzheimer's.[30]

Finally, too much stress or poorly managed stress can also negatively impact the brain both through its direct effects on the brain structures themselves and its indirect effects on other systems like the endocrine system.

General Recommendations for Nervous System Health

Though still not as well understood, various dietary strategies that promote ketosis, like intermittent fasting and Keto, may provide short- and long-term benefits regarding the brain and brain function. Likewise, a plant-based diet high in antioxidant-rich, whole plant foods and healthy fats also promotes brain health. An active lifestyle appears just as important as regular movement keeps the brain healthy and the spinal cord and the peripheral nerves functioning properly.

Finally, adequate sleep is believed to play a critical role in brain health, especially in preventing diseases like Alzheimer's, while dealing with stress goes a long way toward optimal brain function.

Summary

A common mistake people make when trying to shed excess pounds is to choose a nutrition and movement strategy that focuses primarily, if not exclusively, on creating a calorie deficit. Yet, while calories do matter, they are not the only thing that matter. To build a lean, strong, and healthy body, we need to eat and move in ways that support the health of our entire body. Simply counting calories or macros and engaging in sweat fests does not necessarily support the optimal functioning of our organs and body systems. On the other hand, strategies like eating lots of fruits and veggies, limiting added sugars and processed foods, getting adequate sleep, fasting for at least twelve hours, and moving in ways that feel good but that also challenge the body not only support leanness but also support health. What we eat, how we move, and our sleep are not just important when it comes to losing excess weight or achieving our desired body aesthetic. They are critical for promoting a healthy body that radiates health both internally and externally over both the short term and the long term.

BODY IMAGE,
DIET CULTURE,
DISORDERED EATING

I decided to include this section after talking to a colleague who is not only a physical therapist like myself but also a successful online running coach who has worked with thousands of women around the globe, helping them to get leaner, fitter, and stronger.

As experienced healthcare professionals, we have observed that an individual's attitudes about their body, themselves, and their weight as well as how those attitudes affect their relationship with food and movement can be a serious roadblock when it comes to both losing weight (getting leaner) and promoting health.

We are not only living in an unnatural food and movement environment that is at odds with our physiology and biology. We are surrounded by unrealistic and exaggerated images of what a healthy body should look like. Too many of the carefully contrived images that bombard us daily are more caricatures of a body than an honest representation of the human form.

This unrealistic standard of beauty has more than paved the way for several highly profitable industries that make money by making us feel inadequate. The beauty industry with its creams and lotions, the supplement industry with its pills and potions, the diet industry with its fads and quick fixes, and the cosmetic surgical industry with its menu of nips, tucks, needle pricks, and procedures continue to raise the beauty bar.

There have always been standards of beauty defined by the prevailing culture, but never has a standard been so completely disconnected from the natural human condition.

And it is not only harming us mentally—because we can never quite live up to the illusion—but it is also harming us physically because we are striving for some ideal that often does not exist without extreme and/or unhealthy measures.

Even as I write this chapter, famous supermodel Linda Evangelista is suing for a cosmetic procedure gone wrong. She underwent *Cool Sculpting*, a popular fat-freezing alternative to liposuction. She claims she originally had the procedure to spot reduce stubborn areas of fat that she could not lose using exercise or diet. But instead of shrinking the fat as advertised, she claims it caused hard and disfiguring lumps to form under the skin thanks to a rare side effect known as paradoxical adipose hyperplasia. She also claims that future liposuction procedures could not correct the damage.

I share this story to make two points. First, if celebrated supermodels cannot achieve beauty without these types of pricey procedures, what hope do the rest of us regular folk have? Second, almost all procedures, potions, and lotions not only have a financial cost, but they also come with a risk, possibly serious risk.

Yet, this is the current standard of beauty that we often aspire to.

And it goes beyond pricey cosmetic procedures. It continues to fuel a diet culture that has made us fatter and promoted a fitness culture that has less to do with health and fitness and more to do with trying to beat our bodies into a shape that will almost always fall short of the unrealistic standard of the hour.

Many women, and increasingly more men, struggle with an eating disorder. Not necessarily the traditional disorders like anorexia or bulimia—although those are still too prevalent—but a less obvious and more insidious eating disorder in which we are at war not only with food but also with our bodies.

Today's women and even some men are not only abusing food and exercise, but they have developed complex, negative emotions around food, exercise, and around their bodies and themselves.

We no longer know how to eat to nourish and support our bodies. Instead, we have mastered ways to deprive it. And we have reduced exercise to punishment or penance because our distorted image in the mirror cannot live up to our unrealistic expectations.

But if my years in health and fitness have taught me anything worth learning, it is that a healthy body starts on the inside and upstairs. More importantly, until we address our dysfunctional relationship with food, exercise, and ourselves, we will always work against the very thing we say we want: a healthy body that reflects health and natural beauty.

No diet and no exercise program, no matter how well-intentioned, can permanently fix a disordered relationship with this shell that carries us through life or the food we use to fuel it.

The ideal will continue to change, perhaps becoming more unrealistic. We will all age, and there will always be things we dislike about ourselves and our appearance. This does not mean we should not try to change things we do not like but instead understand that physical beauty is not only subjective and superficial, it is transient.

In sharing her story, Linda Evangelista talks about the shame she feels regarding her body. She claims she is so uncomfortable in her own skin that she has isolated herself. She thinks the real problem is a procedure gone wrong, resulting in a few lumps. The reality is far more depressing and concerning. If a beautiful supermodel feels incapable of achieving today's beauty standard and is so traumatized by a few lumps and bumps that it has affected every area of her life, where does that leave the rest of us?

It is not just about getting skinny or lean or even super buff. I mean it might be, but if it is, all I can say is be warned. Healthy is not simply a physical aesthetic or physiological state. It is your mental health. It is the status of your relationships. It is your interactions with the world and your attitudes about yourself.

In short, if you want a healthy body that radiates health, start by developing a healthy relationship with your body in the moment (inside and out)—warts, scars, imperfections, and all. Learn to love yourself unconditionally and stop comparing yourself to an ideal that only exists in the airbrushed spreads of a magazine or a strategically edited ad on the internet. Once you do, the behaviors that support health and leanness become about self-love rather than self-loathing. They originate in respect rather than contempt.

By changing your internal dialogue and the way you think about the process and your body and yourself, you significantly change the dynamic. If you do not, you might achieve short-term success (maybe) but often at a very high cost. And chances are that you still will not be happy.

THE PITFALLS
OF FOCUSING
ON WEIGHT

E very day in my No Excuses group, I see people obsessed with weight. Happy they finally lost a little, discouraged or frustrated that they did not, or wondering what they can do to make it happen sooner than later.

They fixate on their current weight, tie success to a transient and arbitrary weight loss goal, and then employ methods that produce quick weight loss even if not permanent.

Unfortunately, as I have tried to convince you throughout this book, there are significant drawbacks to focusing on weight alone.

For starters, when most people say they want to lose weight, what they really mean is they want to lose fat or become leaner.

However, simply losing weight says nothing about what is contributing to the change on the scale. It might be fat, but it is more likely a combination of fat, water, muscle, and glycogen stores.

A focus on weight also ignores the fact that carrying excess weight (aka excess fat) is a symptom and not the underlying problem.

The underlying problem is the behavior or behaviors that contributed to being overweight/overfat in the first place such as poor eating habits, lack of movement, inadequate sleep, and stress.

Losing weight/fat is tough but keeping it off is almost impossible unless you make real and lasting changes to your daily behaviors, and even then, it can still be tough thanks to the complex physiological feedback loops that contribute to our metabolic function.

Yet still, people are obsessed with those three little numbers. They focus solely on changing the scale, forgetting that getting lean and staying lean requires a real change in lifestyle (our daily choices) and not necessarily the unsustainable and temporary tactics encouraged by most weight-loss, calorie-centered diets/weight-loss programs.

They fail to make the important connection between health, sustainable behavior change, and reaching a desirable and sustainable level of leanness.

Instead of tying their success to behaviors that support a lean, strong, and healthy body over the long term (the focus of this book), they fixate on the scale, unrealistic timelines, and unsustainable methods.

They forget (or just do not realize) that changing behaviors rarely leads to immediate external results, and that there can be a substantial lag between doing the right things and seeing the results we desire.

I often use a garden analogy to illustrate this concept.

Imagine you want to grow a beautiful garden filled with your favorite plants. What that involves may depend on a multitude of factors. For instance, what is the layout of your property? What is the quality of the soil? Is there sufficient light to support the plants you would like to grow? Do you have an old garden that you just need to revamp, or are you starting from scratch? Do you have a piece of land that will be easy to clear, or is it an area filled with invasive plants like poison ivy? Are the plants you want to grow hardy and low maintenance, or do they require prep and upkeep?

Depending on where you are starting and what you hope to grow, it may take considerable effort and hard work before you see the results you are after (beautiful plants growing in your garden). You certainly will not see a plant blooming right away. But this lag in outcome does not reflect a lack of progress. On the contrary, you are making huge gains by doing what is required to lay the foundation for a successful garden long before the garden takes shape.

Sure, you could go to the nursery, buy a flat of healthy plants, stick them in the ground, and throw mulch over the weeds.

Voila...there is your garden.

Or is it?

What feels like progress or immediate success will be short-lived when the weeds pop up through the mulch, and the plants become diseased or fail to thrive in substandard soil conditions. Eventually, all those new plants will wither and die. And this is exactly what happens with most weight loss programs. Quick fixes and diets deliver the illusion of progress, only it rarely lasts, not unless all the other factors needed to support a healthy and lean body over the long term are addressed.

Furthermore, even after you have prepped the lot, addressed the soil, pulled the weeds, and planted the plants, the best-planned gardens will eventually suffer without maintenance.

And so is the case with reaching your health and wellness goals and, specifically, weight loss/leanness goals. You do not simply reach a predetermined and arbitrary number on the scale and then abandon your efforts. You still must tend to the metaphorical garden, although if you have done your prep work well, maintenance should be relatively easy, or at least easier. As is true with the garden analogy, that initial prep time (practicing, internalizing, and eventually mastering those behaviors that support leanness) might not yield immediate returns but they are essential if you hope to achieve lasting results.

The garden analogy demonstrates why fixating on weight is a flawed approach. Weight-centered solutions focus on outcomes (a thriving garden) instead of the process (the work and conditions required to achieve a thriving garden). Real and lasting change requires real and lasting change. Outcomes are linked to the process. Ignore the process or choose one that does not support the long-term results you want, and you will not achieve the long-term results you want, either.

National Weight Control Registry

The National Weight Control Registry, introduced in an earlier section briefly, is an ongoing research project that started back in 1994 to identify behaviors associated with not just losing weight but also with keeping the weight off. By tracking over 10,000 individuals who have lost at least thirty pounds or more and kept it off for at least a year, the researchers have identified several behaviors that appear to correlate with successful long-term weight loss.

The current registry is about 80 percent female and 20 percent male. The average age of women is forty-five years, and the average weight is 145 pounds, while the average age of men is forty-nine years, and the average weight is 190 pounds.

Weight lost ranged from 30 to 300 pounds, while the period for which they maintained the weight loss ranged from one to sixty-six years.

55 percent of registry participants claim they followed a program while the other 45 percent did it on their own.

98 percent of participants altered or changed their eating patterns, while 94 percent increased physical activity. Walking was the most frequently reported activity.

Researchers routinely send participants questionnaires asking about their daily habits. In the data collected, 78 percent reported eating breakfast every day, 75 percent weigh themselves at least once a week, and 90 percent exercise on average one hour a day.[31]

Of course, correlation is not necessarily causation. Simply because two things appear related does not mean they are. But it is certainly worth considering what these participants have in common, which appears to be that they continue to practice behaviors that support their goal.

In my experience, the real secret to not only getting lean and healthy but staying there lies not solely in the methods employed (diet and exercise strategy), but more so on the consistency with which those methods are employed over time (a function of the method's sustainability).

Input equals output.

We all know people who lost weight on any number of diets, from low carb to low fat to calorie restricted to macro balanced to intermittent fasting, while engaging in different forms of fitness, from yoga to walking to running to HIIT or a combination of multiple exercise modes. And we have also seen many of them regain weight once the diet or the challenge is over. But for the few people who lose weight and keep it off, they do so because they make a permanent change to their daily behaviors. And this is where habits come in since our ability to be consistent hinges on adopting behaviors that support a lean, strong, and healthy body not just for the twelve-week fitness challenge but for the rest of our lives.

Again, real and lasting change requires real and lasting change.

Change input temporarily and output may change but only temporarily. But change input permanently and you also change output permanently.

Building habits (input) that support your desired goals (output) is the best way to achieve lasting results.

We are what we repeatedly do. End of story.

PUTTING IT ALL TOGETHER

R eal and lasting change requires real and lasting change. Making real and lasting change takes time. It is rarely straightforward, and it is a slow process dotted with failure.

But it is the only thing that works.

Everything else is the metaphorical band-aid. A quick fix. And yes, just because it took you a year to lose sixty pounds does not mean it is not a quick fix. Anything that does not address long-term behavior in a meaningful and sustainable way is by default a quick fix, regardless of how long it takes.

The fitness/wellness/health journey has no end.

You do not reach some point and get to stop. You must keep going. You must keep acting in ways that support your goals. You must keep tending the metaphorical garden. Health is not permanent, and neither is weight. They are fluid and influenced by our daily choices. That is the bad news, I suppose. There is no finish line to cross, only new ground to cover. The good news is that it is never too late. Each day is an opportunity to make better choices. Each moment and each choice provide us a chance to act in ways that support our desired outcome. It also gets easier, especially when you develop habits that support your goals rather than work against them.

And mindset can be a dealbreaker. Without the right

mindset, not only will most approaches fail, but even if they succeed, the results will often be temporary.

Setting realistic SMART goals that focus on the virtues of progress, process, and practice as opposed to perfection is a good place to start.

Life is a series of challenges and obstacles, which means we must also learn how to weather the inevitable storms we will encounter. But this is also a skill that will get better with time and practice.

I have tried to provide you with the basics of what I have learned over the past thirty years through my formal and informal education, my professional experiences in health, fitness, and wellness, and my own personal health and wellness journey, a journey that has spanned 50-plus years.

The devil really is in the details. It is not the grand gestures, the jaw-dropping transformations. It is the little things that when added together result in big things. Too often people try to change too much too quickly, only it is a poor strategy simply because we are creatures of habit and habit is powerful. And that is the point.

But if we can build habits that support our goals, we can use the power of habit to lift us up rather than weigh us down.

It is okay to think big, but you must start small by slowly mastering the behaviors that support your goals.

The process is slow. Immediate results are not guaranteed. An arbitrary reading on the scale may or may not reflect our effort at any point in time. But anything else misses the root of the problem: our daily choices and our habits.

In this book, we discussed the common mindset flaws and attitudes about the process that can keep you from succeeding. We also discussed common traits shared by those who are successful on this journey both in the short and long term. We covered different eating and movement strategies and explored how they may or may not serve you in pursuit of your goals. Hoping to stress the role of nutrition and exercise as it relates to your health and not just your weight, we briefly examined the various organ systems, their function, and how our choices affect them both directly and indirectly. I shared my own personal strategies (eating seven to eight servings of fruits and veggies a day, limiting added sugar, increasing the overnight fast, moving daily in ways that feel good but also challenge us, getting quality sleep, de-stressing, and learning how to indulge responsibly), explaining why these strategies are effective. We briefly explored important though less understood factors like gut health, food allergies, hormones, and food sensitivities. We touched on several issues that come up repeatedly in my No Excuses group. Topics like motivation, macros, calorie counting, calorie deficits, non-hungry and emotional eating, as well as the role and safety of supplements.

While impossible to whittle down the last thirty years into a book, I have done my best to do just that.

My goal is not to tell you what to do, but to give you the benefit of my experiences so that you can make better-informed choices as you encounter all the conflicting information out there.

Not everyone who reads this book will be ready for its message. The *calorie deficit, sweat fest, scale-centered, carbs are bad, protein powders are necessary, I just need more of the secret ingredient approach* is deeply ingrained in our psyche. The seduction of the magic pill—the quick fix, the too-good-to-be-true promise—is as old as humankind itself.

None of us is completely immune to it.

Yet, we all intuitively know that there is no one-size-fits-all approach to healthy living. What works well for one may fail miserably for another. Thus, finding our sweet spot is part of the challenge, and mapping out our unique journey to our ideal destination is the road that leads to personal success.

Unfortunately, we have made getting healthy and getting lean more complicated than it needs to be. Simple strategies, when mastered and employed consistently, can lead to massive changes that are not only notable but sustainable. No purchase required.

Invest in the process instead of the outcome and the outcome will follow. Focus on the outcome instead of the process and there is no guarantee the outcome will be sustainable.

I hope you close this book with a better understanding of how to build and maintain a lean, strong, and healthy body, and an appreciation for why people fail long term. I also hope that you can approach this journey as a privilege in which self-love and acceptance pave the road to success; that you learn not only how to improve, enhance, and prolong the length of your days, weeks, months, and years on this planet but also the quality of those days, weeks, months, and years. Finally, I hope you focus on building lean, strong, and healthy bodies that serve you well, today, and tomorrow, and for all the tomorrows to follow.

Good Luck and My Warmest, Heartfelt Wishes,

Shaun

[1] NCHS Data Brief, Number 395, December 2020 (cdc.gov)

[2] Economic Costs of Diabetes in the U.S. in 2017 | Diabetes Care | American Diabetes Association (diabetesjournals.org)

[3] https://www.cidrap.umn.edu/news-perspective/2021/04/obesity-studies-highlight-severe-covid-outcomes-even-young-adults

[4] Causes of Obesity | Overweight & Obesity | CDC

[5] Why do dieters regain weight? (apa.org)

[6] Only 1 in 10 Adults Get Enough Fruits or Vegetables | CDC Online Newsroom | CDC

[7] https://www.ewg.org/

[8] https://www.dietaryguidelines.gov

[9] https://www.heart.org

[10] https://www.frontiersin.org/articles/10.3389/fnut.2021.640621/full

[11] 10.1016/j.cub.2015.12.046

[12] National Weight Control Registry (nwcr.ws)

[13] https://www.apa.org

[14] https://www.health.harvard.edu

[15] https://medlineplus.gov

[16] https://onlinelibrary.wiley.com/doi/full/10.1111/acel.13626

[17] https://doi.org/10.1111/acel.13626

[18] 10.1016/j.expneurol.2010.12.007

[19] Science. 2013 Sep 6; 341(6150): 10.1126/science.1241214. doi: 10.1126/science.1241214

[20] Gut microbes affect harmful compound in red meat | National Institutes of Health (NIH)

[21] Calcium supplements and cardiovascular risk: 5 years on - PMC (nih.gov)

[22] Frontiers | The Leptin System and Diet: A Mini Review of the Current Evidence | Endocrinology (frontiersin.org)

[23] Ghrelin | You and Your Hormones from the Society for Endocrinology

[24] Why stress causes people to overeat - Harvard Health

[25] Cortisol: What It Is, Function, Symptoms & Levels (clevelandclinic.org)

[26] History of the ketogenic diet - Wheless - 2008 - Epilepsia - Wiley Online Library

[27] https://www.ncbi.nlm.nih.gov/pmc/articles/PMC6005194/

[28] 2-Deoxy-D-glucose protects hippocampal neurons against excitotoxic and oxidative injury: evidence for the involvement of stress proteins - PubMed (nih.gov)

[29] Yoga Effects on Brain Health: A Systematic Review of the Current Literature - PMC (nih.gov)

[30] Sleep deprivation increases Alzheimer's protein | National Institutes of Health (NIH)

[31] National Weight Control Registry (nwcr.ws)

Made in the USA
Middletown, DE
22 February 2023

25374150R00142